Ann Cowcher is a Senior Tutor at St Bartholomew's School of Nursing, London. She gained a B.A. (Hons) degree in psychology and sociology and Diplomas in Nursing and Nurse Education. She currently holds a place on the Masters course in the Philosophy of Health Care run by Cardiff University.

Shirley Willock is a nurse teacher at St Bartholomew's School of Nursing, teaching student nurses undergoing Registered General Nurse training. She studied for two years in the Department of Nursing at the University of Manchester and gained a Diploma in Advanced Nursing Studies, teaching qualifications for both clinical and classroom teaching and an M.Sc.

Pan Study Aids for GCSE include:

Accounting

Biology

Chemistry

Commerce

Computer Studies

Economics

English Language

French

Geography 1

Geography 2

German

History 1: World History since 1914

History 2: Britain and Europe since 1700

Human Biology

Mathematics

Physics

Sociology

Study Skills

PAN STUDY AIDS

RGN NURSING

Ann Cowcher and Shirley Willock

A Pan Original
Pan Books London, Sydney and Auckland

First published 1988 by Pan Books Ltd,
Cavaye Place, London SW10 9PG

9 8 7 6 5 4 3 2 1

© Ann Cowcher and Shirley Willock

ISBN 0 330 30418 6

Text design by Peter Ward
Text illustration by M L Design
Photoset by Parker Typesetting Service, Leicester
Printed and bound in Spain by
Mateu Cromo SA, Madrid

CONTENTS

Preface   9
Acknowledgements   11

Part One

1 ▶ Introduction   15

2 ▶ The management of nursing care   23

3 ▶ Health and illness   39

4 ▶ The use of research in nursing   55

5 ▶ Ethical and legal issues in nursing practice   81

Part Two

Vignette 1 ▶ Edith and Albert Baker: he has Alzheimer's disease and
is admitted to hospital following an accident at home   99

Vignette 2 ▶ Lisa Barratt has Down's syndrome and is cared for by
her family   104

Vignette 3 ▶ Eric Brown is having treatment for cancer of the lung   110

Vignette 4 ▶ Anne Ellis is an elderly person who collapses at home following a stroke. She needs nutritional advice and follow-up in the community following discharge 116

Vignette 5 ▶ Rosa French, a lady with rheumatoid arthritis, is admitted to hospital for respite care 122

Vignette 6 ▶ Lydia Francis, with multiple sclerosis, is cared for by her husband at home 128

Vignette 7 ▶ Bipti Gopal is admitted to hospital with a ruptured appendix 133

Vignette 8 ▶ Peter Gray has AIDS and is admitted to hospital 137

Vignette 9 ▶ Geoff Lane and Percy Knowles are both admitted to hospital and undergo lower limb amputation 142

Vignette 10 ▶ Charles Lewis is killed in a road traffic accident on his way home from work 147

Vignette 11 ▶ Jonathan London is a teenager who sniffs glue 152

Vignette 12 ▶ Janette and Barry Martins: Janette finds the strain of caring for two small children overwhelming 157

Contents 7

Vignette 13 ▶ Ian Metcalfe fractures a femur and is in hospital for
three months   162

Vignette 14 ▶ Sylvia Norman is experiencing an acute episode
of cystitis   169

Vignette 15 ▶ Angela Poole finds a lump in her breast and seeks
treatment   177

Vignette 16 ▶ Samantha Rice aged 4½ has acute leukaemia   182

Vignette 17 ▶ James Ryder is admitted to hospital with sickle cell crisis   187

Vignette 18 ▶ Mavis Snowden experiences a profound change in
body image because of an endocrine disorder   192

Vignette 19 ▶ George Stevens came into hospital for 'routine' surgery   197

Vignette 20 ▶ Jane Walters chooses to have her pregnancy terminated   202

Vignette 21 ▶ William Watson and Graham Dawson are both admitted
to a cardiac unit in the middle of the night   207

Vignette 22 ▶ Rose Wilkins is dying in hospital   213

Contents

Vignette 23 ▶   **Derek Williams has diabetes mellitus and is too busy to look after his health**   **218**

Index   **222**

PREFACE

We have compiled this Study Guide for nursing students who are undertaking an educational programme leading to registration as a Registered General Nurse. As two teachers of nursing we are used to trying to foster in students the spirit of enquiry necessary to develop, revise and extend the knowledge, skills and attitudes that are needed in order to practise nursing today.

We hope this Study Guide will assist the development of these abilities in its readers. We emphasize here that this book is a study guide rather than a textbook or a revision aid or examination crammer.

The Guide is in two parts. Part One has chapters which focus on the management of nursing care, health and illness, using research in nursing, and ethical and legal issues in nursing practice. Part Two is composed of 'vignettes' in which the situations of particular people who have health problems are explored.

Each chapter and vignette reflects the partial and personal perspective of the authors. We fully acknowledge that the questions we pose, and our guidelines for further study, are not by any means totally comprehensive or all encompassing. This is intentional!

We hope students will, by using this guide, enjoy learning about nursing and will extend the scope of the chapters and vignettes by their own research and study. The margins are deliberately wide to allow space for students to add their own references and notes, and in Chapter 1 we make suggestions about developing personal information resources which will help the student with this process.

We have deliberately used a small number of well-known textbooks and journals which are very likely to be found in School of Nursing libraries. These are cited in brief in the text, and can be found in full at the end of each chapter under the 'References' heading. These sources have limitations, of course, and we strongly advise students to adopt a critical stance towards the references given, and to use other textbooks and journals which they may prefer and which may also be available to them. Our intention is to motivate students actively to seek out and develop their own knowledge sources, not so much making a guide like this superfluous but rather helping further towards creating and developing in nurses the necessary spirit of enquiry.

In other words, a student nurse working his or her way through this book, or simply dipping into it and considering individual chapters and vignettes will, we hope, have been signposted towards some of the possible directions in which he or she can enquire further. Nursing students will already be guided by their teachers towards developing what is held by the profession to be the necessary knowledge, skills and attitudes for practice as a nurse. We can only hope to become another resource for students to draw upon.

ACKNOWLEDGEMENTS

We have been greatly influenced by colleagues, students and teachers, throughout our careers, and particularly recently by those at St Bartholomew's School of Nursing. Our involvement there with the revision of the curriculum and its translation into practice has been a keystone. We owe a debt of gratitude and respect for these colleagues and this influence. In addition we offer grateful thanks to our families and friends who have kept us sane.

Our thanks, too, to Mr T. Keighley, Director of Nursing, Waltham Forest Health Authority, for reading and reporting favourably on our typescript.

PART ONE

INTRODUCTION

CONTENTS

▶ **The competencies of a registered nurse**   17
The curriculum   17

▶ **Studying nursing**   19
Finding out   19
Personal study resources   20

▶ **Using this study guide**   21
The chapters and vignettes   21
Textbooks and journals   22

▶ **References**   22

THE COMPETENCIES OF A REGISTERED NURSE

THE CURRICULUM

At the time of writing, in the late 1980s, nursing education in the United Kingdom is hopefully on the threshold of profound change. Recent analyses of the education of students of nursing (RCN 1985, ENB 1985, UKCC 1986) have pointed yet again to the need to give all nursing students an educational preparation for nursing before they are employed to nurse people and become part of the nursing workforce. This preparation of theory and closely supervised practice will ensure that they have the knowledge and skills to nurse people before they take on and carry responsibilities for doing so.

Until this change takes place, except in a few pilot schemes and undergraduate programmes, nursing students are employees and form part of the nursing service given to patients. They undergo their formal education as they nurse patients and during study days and weeks.

The education programme students undergo and the assessments they have to complete in order to be able to become a Registered General Nurse, are overseen and agreed by the National Boards. The Boards provide broad curriculum guidelines and each School of Nursing develops its own programme of education and assessment.

The resulting individualized nature of the programmes and assessment strategies does, though, have a single goal: it must enable the nursing student to develop the essential competencies of a Registered Nurse. These competencies are to:

advise on the promotion of health and the prevention of illness;

recognize situations that may be detrimental to the health and well-being of the individual;

carry out those activities involved when conducting the comprehensive assessment of a person's nursing requirements;

recognize the significance of the observations made and use these to develop an initial nursing assessment;

devise a plan of nursing care based on the assessment with the co-operation of the patient, to the extent that this is possible, taking into account the medical prescription;

implement the planned programme of nursing care and, where appropriate, teach and co-ordinate other members of the caring team who may be responsible for implementing specific aspects of the nursing care;

review the effectiveness of the nursing care provided and, where appropriate, initiate any action that may be required;

work in a team with other nurses, and with medical and para-medical staff and social workers;

undertake the management of the care of a group of patients over a period of time and organize the appropriate support services.

These competencies, which are stated in *The Nurses, Midwives and Health Visitors Rules Approval Order* 1983 (Statutory Instrument 1983, No. 873) HMSO London, are used as a framework for this Study Guide. In addition we have taken account of the other 'competencies' outlined in Project 2000 (UKCC, 1986) since they probably indicate the direction towards which curriculum development is progressing:

demonstrate knowledge and skills necessary to meet the health and sickness requirements of individuals and of groups in a particular area of practice;

recognise common factors which contribute to and those which adversely effect physical, mental and social well-being of patients or clients and take appropriate action;

identify the social and health implications of physical and mental handicap or disease, and pregnancy and childbearing, for the individual, his or her friends, family and community;

demonstrate knowledge of the normal development of the foetus, the infant, the child, the adolescent and the young, middle-aged and elderly adult;

demonstrate an appreciation of research and use relevant literature and research as an aid to practice;

demonstrate professional accountability and commitment to continuing professional education and development;

demonstrate an awareness of social and political factors which relate to health care;

demonstrate knowledge and understanding to meet the requirements of legislation which is relevant to her practice;

recognize and uphold the confidential rights of patients and clients;

develop helpful caring relationships with patients, clients and their families or friends; initiate, continue and complete therapeutic relationships with patients using appropriate interpersonal and communication skills;

identify health-related learning needs of patients, clients, family or friends and participate in health promotion;

demonstrate an awareness of the roles of individual members of the team who provide aspects of patient/client care, function efficiently in a team and assist in a multidisciplinary approach where appropriate;

assign appropriate work to helpers and provide supervision and monitoring of assigned work;

identify physical, psychological, social and spiritual needs of the patient or client; be aware of and value the concept of individual care, and devise a plan of care, contribute to its implementation and evaluation by demonstrating an appreciation and practice of the problem solving approach;

enable patients or clients as appropriate to progress from varying degrees of dependence to maximal independence, or to a peaceful death.

STUDYING NURSING

FINDING OUT

Perhaps you already know how to do this! If you are not sure, read on for a selection of suggestions.

What is your principal interest in life at the moment? What strategy are you using in order to develop that interest?

Is the strategy similar to the way in which you are pursuing your interest in your chosen occupation, nursing?

CONSULTING OTHER PEOPLE

Your strategy is likely to include the idea of consulting people with experience and expertise. Using this strategy in order to study nursing is important, and fellow students, qualified nurses, teachers and library staff are obvious examples of such people.

CONSULTING WRITTEN MATERIALS

Another way is to consider some of the written material that is available, and to use libraries. You were introduced to the library facilities in your School of Nursing as soon as you started your nursing course. However, it is possible that unless you have had to use actively the information you were given at that time you may be rather uncertain about it now! The best way of acquiring this essential skill of finding out information using library resources is by practising it; seek out information and use the expertise the librarian has to offer.

Your School of Nursing library will have a system of cataloguing the books and journals that it holds. Make sure you develop your confidence in using it. Your library will hold a variety of bibliographies and indexing and abstracting journals. They will list published material under subject headings. The books and journals to which they refer may not be available in your library, but the librarian may be able to acquire them for you.

Try this exercise: locate the nursing bibliographies and abstracting and indexing journals in your School of Nursing library, and use them to find material on a chosen subject such as wound care, pain relief or incontinence.

Whilst in the library check with your librarian whether he or she has organized card index files of books and articles under similar subject headings.

One systematic way of finding out information is by carrying out a literature search. Some useful guidelines are found in Pollock (1984), Sheehan (1985) and Kwater (1987).

REFLECTING ON YOUR PERSONAL EXPERIENCE

The remainder of your strategy for further developing your interest in a topic, in addition to using the expertise and experience of people, and investigating written materials, is likely to be by using your personal knowledge and experiences. You will find that throughout this Guide you will be asked to reflect back on your personal experiences, and you will be asked to think about what you have learned from them.

Your own experience is valuable. You may find it helpful, whilst studying nursing, to record your personal experiences of caring for patients alongside your lecture notes and the study notes you make when reading. This personal knowledge of nursing practice helps you estimate the value and see the relevance of the theoretical knowledge you are developing.

PERSONAL STUDY RESOURCES

In addition to your personal strategy for studying and for developing your interest in nursing you need to think about how you could develop your own easily accessible sources of information. What about reconsidering the textbooks you have? Do you use them, do you even like them? Have you come across books in the library which you would prefer to have? One way round this may be to exchange or sell them and acquire the books you really would like to have by you and which you will find useful.

You will find that reading journals is a productive way of studying and updating your knowledge.

In using this Guide you will read many articles from nursing journals. In locating these articles you will come across others which interest you. Get into the habit of noting down the exact reference for the article in a notebook or on index cards so that you can find the article again.

As you develop your interest in a topic, for example wound care, pain relief or incontinence, you can develop and update your notes or take further photocopies. By developing and refining your areas of interest you will find that your reading becomes easier because you will know what you want to get out of a journal and need only skim through it.

In addition to physically gathering books and photocopied articles around you, you can develop a personal system of keeping notes about areas of interest using notebooks or index cards. With index cards, this involves writing the full title of the article or chapter you have read on the index card with a short summary of its key points. The index cards can be kept by you in boxes under separate headings, and if necessary you can then refer back to the original source easily when you need to.

USING THIS STUDY GUIDE

THE CHAPTERS AND VIGNETTES

In the Preface to this Guide we have stated that the contents of the chapters and the vignettes do not 'cover' the entire scope of the subjects they address. The content could have been different and we could have explored the topics in other ways. By acknowledging this we hope to motivate you to take an active part in developing the content of the Guide for yourselves. By doing this you will focus on the dimensions that interest you and you will extend the breadth and depth of the content.

In each chapter and vignette we have separated out and highlighted the essential activities which we would like, from this distance, to urge you to try out, and we have made some suggestions for your further study at the end of each one.

We have not focused on anatomy, physiology or pathology to any great extent. This has been deliberate. This does not mean that these subjects are not important and that nurses do not need to study them, but rather that we have not chosen to focus on them here. We know you will be developing your knowledge in these areas in the educational pro-gramme you are undertaking anyway. But, if knowledge of anatomy, physiology and pathology is essential for understanding some of the problems of the patient in certain vignettes we have made this clear in the activities at the beginning.

The chapters in Part One form a foundation for some of the study activities in Part Two and also provide an overview of some of the theory underlying nursing practice as outlined in the competencies (pages 17 and 18). We suggest you read through the whole of Part One before embarking on Part Two.

In Part Two, in the vignettes, a person with a health problem is focused on. The vignette begins with references and suggested topics for you to investigate. Space has been left for you to write in other references which you find helpful. The description of a person with a health problem then follows with a number of activities for you to undertake. When you have completed the activities you will have built up an understanding of that health problem.

You will find that the characters in the vignettes usually have only one or two health problems. We know and accept that this is somewhat unrealistic. Our experience and that of our students is that people, more often than not, have a number of health problems and also face complex and difficult situations. However, we have chosen to focus on people with only one or two health problems in order to separate them out and put them into a manageable form for studying.

TEXTBOOKS AND JOURNALS

The principal textbooks that we have referred to in the Guide are:

Ellison Nash, D. F. 1980. *The Principles and Practice of Surgery for Nurses.* 7th edition. Edward Arnold, London.

Faulkner, A. 1985. *Nursing. A Creative Approach.* Baillière Tindall, London.

Houston, J. C., Joiner, C.L. and Trounce, J.R. 1982. *A Short Textbook of Medicine.* 7th edition. Hodder and Stoughton, London.

Macleod, J. (Editor) 1981. *Davidson's Principles and Practice of Medicine.* 13th edition. Churchill Livingstone, Edinburgh.

Roper, N., Logan, W.W. and Tierney, A.J. 1985. *The Elements of Nursing.* 2nd edition. Churchill Livingstone, Edinburgh.

Watson, J. E. and Royle, J.R. 1987. *Watson's Medical-Surgical Nursing and Related Physiology.* 3rd edition. Baillière Tindall, London.

Wilson, K. J. W. 1987. *Ross and Wilson. Anatomy and Physiology in Health and Illness.* 6th edition. Churchill Livingstone, Edinburgh.

The journals we have used extensively are *Nursing Mirror*, *Nursing Times*, *Journal of Advanced Nursing* and *Nursing* (the Add-On Journal of Clinical Nursing). N.B. We have used the British, not the US, journal of this name.

REFERENCES TO CHAPTER 1

English National Board. 1985. *Professional Education Training Courses.* Consultation Paper. ENB. London.

Kwater, S. 1987. Literature searching for starters. *Nurse Education Today*, Vol.7, No.3. June, pp.132–4.

Pollock, L. 1984. Six steps to a successful literature search. *Nursing Times*, 31 October, pp.40–43.

RCN. 1985. *The Education of Nurses: A New Dispensation.* (The Judge Report) RCN, London.

Sheehan, J. 1985. Reviewing the literature. *Nursing Mirror*, 8 May, pp.29–30.

UKCC. 1986. *Project 2000. A New Preparation for Practice.* UKCC, London.

THE MANAGEMENT OF NURSING CARE

CONTENTS

The nature of nursing 26
Models of nursing 26
The concept of nursing 27

The nursing process 30
Assessment 31
Planning 32
Implementation 32
Evaluation 33

Delivering nursing care 33
Patient allocation 33
Task allocation 33
Team nursing 33
Primary nursing 33

Measuring the quality of nursing care 34
Quality assurance programmes 35
The politics of nursing 36

Further study 36

References 36

Five of the competencies of a nurse are to:

Carry out those activities involved when conducting the comprehensive assessment of a person's nursing requirements.

Recognize the significance of the observations made and use these to develop an initial nursing assessment.

Devise a plan of nursing care based on the assessment with the co-operation of the patient, to the extent that this is possible, taking into account the medical prescription.

Implement the planned programme of nursing care and, where appropriate, teach and co-ordinate other members of the caring team who may be responsible for implementing specific aspects of the nursing care.

Review the effectiveness of the nursing care provided and, where appropriate, initiate any action that may be required.

In this chapter we will consider the ways in which a patient's needs for nursing can be met.

The competencies outlined above reflect the way in which nursing care is decided upon, shared with others, carried out and evaluated. As nurses we are required to make written recordings of this decision-making process by the organization in which we work. These records help in the relaying of information and instructions about a patient's nursing care to other members of the nursing team, and they can serve as evidence of the care given.

A fundamental feature of present-day nursing practice is to give care which is individualized and meets the unique needs of each person cared for. But, at the same time, such ideal practice is constrained by the resources which are available; the skills the nursing team possesses, the time that is available, the facilities and equipment to hand and, of course, the 'amount' of nursing care our patients need.

In this chapter the nature of nursing and its reflection in 'models of nursing' is touched on, together with an overview of the 'nursing process'. Some of the systems of organizing the work of nurses are outlined too.

At the end of the chapter a very brief outline is given of some of the strategies for measuring the quality of nursing care.

THE NATURE OF NURSING

MODELS OF NURSING

A nursing model or conceptual framework is a representation of what nursing is believed, in certain situations, to be. Nursing models appear as written statements and sometimes as diagrams. They describe nursing and those who are nursed, and the way the activities of nurses and patients interact and are directed.

Nurses who develop such models attempt to analyse the many activities of nurses and patients, and try to make some sense of how they fit together. They take care to analyse each part of their model, each abstract concept which is being manipulated.

One example of linking abstract concepts which can clarify some ideas about nursing is illustrated by McFarlane and Castledine (1982). The authors show, by the aid of a simple diagram, the way in which nursing is linked with the concepts of man, society and health.

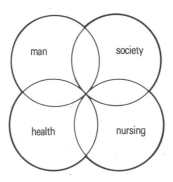

Another well-known example of linking different concepts is that of the decision-making strategy used in determining how to nurse a patient, the nursing process. This links the four activities of assessment, planning, implementation and evaluation. A number of diagrammatic permutations are possible, for example:

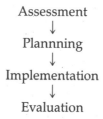

Assessment
↓
Plannning
↓
Implementation
↓
Evaluation

This one implies that the process is carried out by completing the individual steps in a linear fashion. Another representation of the nursing process could be:

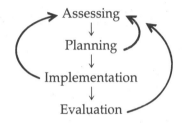

This diagram shows that the steps of the nursing process are inter-linked and affect each other, and that the process may proceed in a number of possible directions.

If you were to develop a model of nursing you would attempt to go further than simply linking concepts. You would, for example, be more specific about what nurses need to assess in patients they are nursing. You would try to answer a number of questions which might include what has to be assessed and why, whether or not it is indeed possible to assess the items chosen, and whether any tools are available to help you.

In building such a model you would also attempt to make explicit those activities which would need to be planned in order to meet the patient's needs, those revealed during their nursing assessment, and would propose how those activities could be implemented and evaluated.

A useful series of articles about nursing models has been produced by Peter Aggleton and Helen Chalmers and published in the *Nursing Times*:

1   Models and theories and Johnson's behavioural systems model   5 September 1984, pp.24–8.
2   Roy's adaptation model   3 October 1984, pp.45–8.
3   Riehl's interaction model   7 November 1984, pp.58–61.
4   Roger's unitary field model   12 December 1984, pp.35–9.
5   Orem's self-care model   2 January 1985, pp.36–9.
6   Roper's activities of living model   13 February 1985, pp.59–61.
7   Henderson's model   6 March 1985, pp.33–5.
8   Critical examination   3 April 1985, pp.38–9.

In addition the authors have written a book: Aggleton and Chalmers 1986.

However, before devising your model you must formulate a clear definition of nursing. You could then go on to propose specific details about assessment, planning, implementation and evaluation.

THE CONCEPT OF NURSING

Nursing is a difficult concept to pin down, and any definitions will reflect the beliefs and values held by those who make them.

Think about, and write down, your own definition of the concept of nursing. What is nursing?

Compare your definition and ideas with those included in McFarlane and Castledine 1982, Aggleton and Chalmers 1984/5 (see above); see also nursing textbooks in your library which give a definition of nursing.

One well-known statement made about the nature of nursing and the function of the nurse is that of the American nurse, Virginia Henderson (1966, p.15): 'The unique function of the nurse is to assist the individual, sick or well, in the performance of those activities contributing to health or its recovery (or to a peaceful death) that he would perform unaided if he had the necessary strength, will or knowledge. And to do this in such a way as to help him gain independence as rapidly as possible.'

Henderson maintains that nursing activities are directed towards enabling the patient to become 'self-caring'. In circumstances when the patient is unable to care for himself because of illness she acknowledges that nurses may need to act for, and instead of, the patient. Nurses take part in and help facilitate the medical treatment of the patient, and the nurse co-ordinates, on behalf of the patient, the activities of the other professionals who are involved in his care.

Nursing activities, according to Henderson, are directed towards helping the patient to fulfil what are described as 'the activities of daily living'. These activities enable the patient to:

1   Breathe normally.
2   Eat and drink adequately.
3   Eliminate body wastes.
4   Move and maintain desirable postures.
5   Sleep and rest.
6   Select suitable clothes – dress and undress.
7   Maintain body temperature within normal range by adjusting clothing and modifying the environment.
8   Keep the body clean and well groomed and protect the integument.
9   Avoid danger in the environment and avoid injuring others.
10 Communicate with others in expressing emotions, needs, fear or opinions.
11 Worship according to one's faith.
12 Work in such a way that there is a sense of accomplishment.
13 Play or participate in various forms of recreation.
14 Learn, discover or satisfy the curiosity that leads to normal development and health and use the available health facilities.

In the United Kingdom Roper, Logan and Tierney (1981, 1983a, 1985) have described twelve 'activities of living'. These activities are similar to Henderson's, but they also include the activities of 'expressing sexuality' and 'dying':

1   Maintaining a safe environment.
2   Communicating.
3   Breathing.
4   Eating and drinking.
5   Eliminating.

6   Personal cleansing and dressing.
7   Controlling body temperature.
8   Mobilizing.
9   Working and playing.
10 Expressing sexuality.
11 Sleeping.
12 Dying.

There are many easily accessible books and articles written about Roper *et al.*'s approach to nursing. Some of the key ideas appear in the article Roper, Logan and Tierney (1983b).

Roper *et al.*, in their model of nursing, propose that nurses need to assess their patients' abilities to carry out the activities of living (A.L.s). This assessment should take into account the patients' level of independence in managing the activities of living for themselves before illness, their level of independence during illness, and the potential problems likely to occur in their ability to carry out activities of living in the future in response to their ill health.

The authors stress, and it will be clear to you when nursing, that each of the activities of living is affected by a person's individual social and economic circumstances, his cultural and religious background and his individual psychological and physiological responses to situations.

Orem (1980, p.56), an American nurse, also sees nursing as an 'assisting' and 'helping' service. She draws attention to the skilled nature of this assisting and helping, and makes the following claim: 'Although the tasks performed may be quite simple, it is complicated for one person to do something that another person cannot do, must not do, or prefers not to do. It is complicated because the need being met is a requirement of another person.'

This statement of Orem's may reflect something you have found to be true.

1   What are the difficulties you have encountered in trying to 'assist' and 'help' patients?

2   Do you think nursing necessitates something in addition to assisting and helping people?

Both Henderson and Orem view the patient as recovering his own health or achieving a peaceful death with the assistance of the nurse.

THE NURSE–PATIENT RELATIONSHIP

Ujhely (1968) adds a further dimension to the concept of the nurse assisting or helping the patient, that of 'sustaining' the patient through the experience of being ill. She sees this sustenance being given by the nurse to the patient by means of their developing relationship.

This nurse-patient relationship is held to be of great importance in nursing. Sundeen *et al.* (1981) explore the relationship in some depth and consider the concepts of trust, empathy, autonomy and mutuality in the relationship, together with the dimension of caring or love.

The authors draw on the work of Rogers (1961) to illustrate the characteristics of such a 'helping relationship'. The relationship is based on three fundamental characteristics of the helping person, the nurse. Firstly, the helper needs to be 'open' and 'genuine' in the relationship with the other person. Secondly, the helper needs to try to achieve an empathic understanding of what the other person is feeling. And thirdly, the helper needs to 'prize' the other person, and hold him in positive regard.

The characteristics of the helper in the nurse/patient relationship are related to one of the fundamental ethical principles used in nursing – that of respect for persons.

INDIVIDUALIZED CARE

An important belief currently held in nursing, and underlying nursing practice, is that nursing should be focused on meeting the individual needs of people. Nursing aims to acknowledge fully the uniqueness and individuality of patients. Nurses try to maintain this individuality even though patients usually have to relate to many different nurses and healthcare workers. For further information on the importance of the individual, see, for example; Kitson 1987.

Beliefs held about the nature of nursing are explored from a sociological perspective in Katherine Williams (1974). She explores three different ideologies of nursing – Vocation, Profession and Custodialism. This article appears, along with other authors' sociological explorations of the occupation of nursing, in Dingwall and McIntosh (1978).

THE NURSING PROCESS

The 'nursing process' is a term used to describe the way in which decisions are made about a person's need for nursing care and how best to provide that care. These decisions are made using a systematic problem-solving strategy. Details vary, but in essence four stages can be identified as making up the process of nursing:

1 Assessment Carrying out a nursing assessment of the patient and documenting it.

2 Planning Making decisions about the patient's 'problems' and producing a written action plan.

3 Implementation Nursing the patient.

4 Evaluation Continually evaluating the nursing given and making written recordings.

Assessing and evaluating are more or less continuous processes. Nurses in hospital and in the community need to adhere to an agreed format and meet local requirements about the written records.

Critically evaluate the documentation used in the hospital or community placement you are currently working in. Direct your evaluation along these lines:

1   Do you consider that the nurses who designed your local documents based them on a known model of nursing? If not, what do the documents reflect about the nature of nursing?
2   What information would you like to record that is not asked for on the form?
3   Would you add to or take away some of the headings on the form if you were in a position to redesign it?
4   Is there a committee or a working party in your hospital or district which might welcome your suggestions for amendments or your positive comments?

ASSESSMENT

This stage of the nursing process includes both the collection of background information about the patient, for example, age, marital status and home address, together with a nursing assessment of the patient which can serve as a basis for making decisions about the nursing he or she will need. It is commonly the case that the nursing assessment is constrained by the 'forms' used in hospitals or the community. The form is likely to reflect, to some extent, the philosophy of nursing held by the nurses who designed the form. It may have many headings to direct what is to be assessed, or it may be blank and require you to formulate what will be assessed.

Assessment takes into account the physical, psychological, social and spiritual needs of the patient. The patient's problems may be actual or potential ones, and some authors refer to the problems as nursing diagnoses (Yura and Walsh 1978).

The assessment pinpoints the problems being experienced by the patient. You will have to determine the priorities of care needed by the patient both in terms of the patient's and the professionals' priorities.

The interpersonal exchanges which take place during the nursing assessment enable the foundation of the nurse–patient relationship to be laid down and ideally it should begin the patient's involvement in his or her care.

Putting aside the possible limitations of the form you use locally to record the nursing assessment, what is your opinion about the actual process of assessing patients in wards and departments in which you have worked?

What are the strengths and weaknesses of the process that you have encountered? How, in particular, could those weaknesses and limitations be overcome?

PLANNING

This stage involves planning the behaviour of both the patient and the nurse in order to reach specific attainable goals. Nursing care is planned to meet priorities of care and is aimed towards achieving goals that, where possible, need to be made explicit and measurable. Goals may be long-term or short-term. The care plan specifies the patient's and/or the nurse's activities which are directed towards reaching the goals of care. Above all, and in most circumstances, the nurse and the patient need to agree the goals of care.

Lewis (1976) suggested the use of 'initial planning options' for common patient problems. This would involve the use of locally agreed and formulated nursing actions for given patient problems. Thus for a problem such as breathlessness, a number of workable action plans would be available to the nurse planning care. She could choose to try out some of the strategies suggested and see if they work. This, it is believed, would help to build up nursing knowledge and focus on areas which need to be investigated.

Three British nurses have written a useful book which focuses on patients' problems, i.e. problems associated with breathing, eating, drinking, sleeping, mobility, religion and social role, and have identified action plans to meet them. See Barnett, Knight and Mabbott 1987.

The care plan is usually handwritten for each patient and may be so specific that it cannot be used for any other patient. In some situations care plans may also incorporate some pre-printed standard instructions and goals for patients who have certain nursing diagnoses. The patient's care plan may then be 'individualized' by means of handwritten instructions to meet the patient's individual needs, over and above what may 'routinely' be required in his or her treatment and care. Mayers (1978) describes the development of standard pre-printed care plans.

In order to implement a care plan you must work out a time schedule which allows for the care of several patients over a span of duty. In addition, Yura and Walsh (1978) identify 'vertical planning' in order to time specific activities. This vertical planning takes into account basic human needs, the patient's circadian rhythms, and promotes the co-ordination of the activities of other health care workers caring for the patient.

IMPLEMENTATION

In this stage of the nursing process the care plan is put into action, and the patient is nursed in such a way as to have the best possible chance of reaching the goals that have been set by both nurse and patient.

Whilst implementing care the nurse observes and reassesses the patient's needs, and is continually solving problems and critically evaluating the care that is being given.

EVALUATION

This is a continuous process. It is closely linked to the process of assessment and goal setting. Care may be formally evaluated at the end of each span of duty or specific aspects of care may be formally evaluated on specified 'review' dates.

Efforts are being made in this country to evaluate nursing care and monitor its quality. This is accomplished by means of analysing or 'auditing' nursing records. (For further discussion, see page 35.)

DELIVERING NURSING CARE

PATIENT ALLOCATION

This is sometimes termed 'total patient care'. In many hospital wards it is customary for the care of individual patients to be allocated to specific nurses over a period of a span of duty. A nurse may continue to care for the same group of patients on subsequent spans of duty or she may be asked to care for a different group. It may be more satisfying for both patient and nurse if the former situation is the case.

TASK ALLOCATION

On occasions it may be necessary for nurses to be allocated tasks associated with patients' care rather than the total care of individual patients. The allocation of such tasks reflects the skills held by the nurse involved. This style of managing the nursing care of patients is said to be necessary when staffing levels are low, and when the range of skills of the whole nursing team of qualified and unqualified persons needs to be channelled in this way for the immediate safety and benefit of patients.

Task allocation may cause problems and concerns for nurses and patients alike. What do *you* think of task allocation? (See Merchant 1985.)

TEAM NURSING

The nursing of patients can be accomplished by setting up teams of nurses and allocating specific groups of patients to their care. A team may be responsible for a geographical area of the ward, or a particular span of duty. It is usual for the team leader to be a qualified nurse, and the team members to be a mixture of qualified nurses, nursing students and untrained personnel.

PRIMARY NURSING

This method of managing nursing care was originally conceptualized and written about in the United States. It is now used in an increasing number of nursing settings in the United Kingdom and there is now accessible literature on its use in this country. (For US texts, see Marram, Barrett and Bevis 1979; Manthey 1980 and Hegyvary 1982. For UK literature, see Pearson 1983, Wright 1987 and Tutton 1987.)

The key feature of primary nursing is that a patient is assigned on admission to a specific qualified nurse. The nurse assesses the patient and plans and evaluates his or her care. Whilst on duty the nurse cares for the patient and in the nurse's absence the care is given by an 'associate nurse' who follows through the 'primary nurse's' care plans.

Thus the primary nurse takes on continuous responsibility for the whole of the patient's stay in hospital. She may also take up and maintain links with the patient on discharge and on subsequent admissions. The primary nurse will have a caseload of her own specific patients, and will also, usually, act as an associate nurse for other primary nurses and their patients.

Reflect back on your recent ward and community experience.

1   How was the nursing care managed in those placements; by task allocation, patient allocation, team nursing or primary nursing, or a mixture?

2   How could the care have been managed, in your estimation, in order to gain the greatest satisfaction for both patients and nurses?

3   In which of your ward or community placements would primary nursing be a viable option for managing patient care?

MEASURING THE QUALITY OF NURSING CARE

Just as we noted at the beginning of this chapter that it is difficult to be precise about the nature of nursing, it is also equally difficult to pin down just what constitutes high quality nursing care.

Select a patient you are currently nursing;

1   Make a list of all the criteria you would take into account if you were trying to decide whether the standard of nursing care given to your patient is below standard, satisfactory or of high quality.

2   What do you consider to be the factors which affect the quality of nursing care?

In general, attempts to measure the quality of patient care focus on three major areas:

The structure The context in which the care takes place. It takes into account factors such as the number of staff available, their educational preparation and qualifications and their nursing experience, together with the facilities available in the work environment for both patients and nurses.

The process What is actually done to the patient. Attempts to measure the process of care will take into account what care is actually received by the patient and how it is administered by nurses; their nursing practice and their interpersonal skills.

The outcome The effect on the health and ill health of the patient as a result of the nursing care received.

In measuring the quality of nursing care the nurse and what she does may be observed at the time the care is given (concurrent assessment of the process). Alternatively, the effects on patients of that nursing care may be focused on – the outcome of care. Nursing records may also be evaluated or audited, as it is termed, at the time the patient is actively being nursed (concurrent audit) or after the patient has been discharged (retrospective audit).

Inman (1975) reports early efforts made in the United Kingdom to pinpoint factors which are important in determining the quality of nursing care. These factors included pre-operative fasting, pain control, nasogastric feeding, the emotional support of children in hospital, admission procedures and dressing techniques.

QUALITY ASSURANCE PROGRAMMES

A number of health authorities in the United Kingdom are developing quality assurance programmes whereby attempts are made to determine and establish standards for specific aspects of nursing care. Subsequently, efforts are made to set up the means to assess whether those agreed standards for patients' nursing care are actually being met. This may be done by observing the care given to patients and also by considering the care recorded in nursing records.

For example, a hospital might determine a specific standard concerning pressure sore prevention in elderly patients. This might involve specifying at what time following admission an initial nursing assessment should be made of patients, how the assessment should be recorded and what actions should be planned to follow. Checks on the care given to patients could then be made concurrently or retrospectively. An evaluation could then be made as to whether the nursing care given met the agreed standard or not.

The original literature on quality assurance programmes is American, but the United Kingdom experience is also on record now. For US literature, see especially Froebe and Bain 1976. Also, for descriptions of measuring the quality of nursing care, see Slater 1967, Phaneuf 1972 and Wandelt and Ager 1974. For UK literature, see Wright 1984, Kitson 1986 and Pearson 1987.

THE POLITICS OF NURSING

At the beginning of this chapter your attention was drawn to some of the constraints within which nurses try to care for patients. Whatever high ideals of care you seek to obtain you will find that you can achieve only so much, given the personnel and facilities that are available. Debate about these difficulties is aired in the nursing literature under the heading 'the politics of nursing'. Good introductory books on this topic are Salvage (1985) and Clay (1987).

FURTHER STUDY

WRITING CARE PLANS IN PART TWO

As you work your way through the vignettes in Part Two you will be called upon to write out care plans for some of the patients whose care is being discussed. Here are some suggestions about how you could do this.

1   You may like to use a care plan format with which you are familiar. Some students are used to writing plans using separate columns for the problem, the goal of care, the actions required, with extra columns to indicate the review dates.
2   Alternatively, you may like to make notes in a less formal manner about the care the patient requires.
3   You may like to experiment by using the format of assessment sheets and care plans you come across in books or journals.

If you feel rather uncertain about the way to write care plans, the following books will give you useful guidelines: McFarlane and Castledine 1982 and Hunt and Marks-Maran 1986.

SUPPORT WORKERS

One of Project 2000's proposals was that nurses should be helped by an assistant, originally referred to as an 'aide'. This helper would be closely supervised by a qualified nurse and would be trained to give a limited range of care for patients. Can you find in the nursing press the current arguments being used in the debate about the role and scope of work undertaken by this worker in the care team? A useful starting point will be Dickson and Cole (1987).

REFERENCES

Aggleton, P. and Chalmers, H. 1984/1985. Series of articles about nursing models. *Nursing Times.* See page 27 for details.

Aggleton, P. and Chalmers, H. 1986. *Nursing Models and the Nursing Process.* Macmillan Education, London.

Barnett, D. E., Knight, G. and Mabbott, A. 1987. *Patients, Problems and*

Plans. Nursing Care of Patients with Medical Disorders. Edward Arnold, London.

Clay, T. 1987. Nurses, power and politics. Heinemann Nursing. London.

Dickson, N. and Cole, A. 1987. Nurses little helper. *Nursing Times.* 11 March, pp.24–6.

Dingwall, R. and McIntosh, J. 1978. *Readings in the Sociology of Nursing.* Churchill Livingstone, Edinburgh.

Froebe, D. J. and Bain, R. J. 1976. *Quality Assurance Programmes and Controls in Nursing.* Mexby, St Louis.

Hegyvary, S. T. 1982. *The Change to Primary Nursing.* C. V. Mosby Co., St Louis.

Henderson, V. 1966. *The Nature of Nursing.* Collier-Macmillan, London.

Hunt, J. M. and Marks-Maran, D. 1986. *Nursing Care Plans: the Nursing Process at Work.* 2nd edition. HM+M Publishers; John Wiley and Sons, London.

Inman, U. 1975. *Towards a Theory of Nursing Care.* RCN, London.

Kitson, A. 1986. The methods of measuring quality. *Nursing Times.* 27 August, pp.27–34.

Kitson, A. 1987. A comparative analysis of lay-caring and professional (nursing) caring relationships. *International Journal of Nursing Studies.* 24 February, pp.155–65.

Lewis, L. 1976. *Planning Patient Care.* 2nd edition. William C. Brown Co., Iowa.

McFarlane, J. K. M. and Castledine, G. 1982. *A Guide to the Practice of Nursing Using the Nursing Process.* C. V. Mosby, London.

Manthey, M. 1980. *The Practice of Primary Nursing.* Blackwell Scientific Publications, Boston.

Marram, G., Barrett, M. W. and Bevis, E. O. 1979. *Primary Nursing. A Model for Individualized Care.* C. V. Mosby Co., St Louis.

Mayers, M. G. 1978. *A Systematic Approach to the Nursing Care Plan.* 2nd edition. Appleton-Century–Crofts, New York.

Merchant, J. 1985. Organising nursing care. Why task allocation? *Nursing Practice*, 1 February, pp.67–71.

Orem, D. 1980. *Nursing: Concepts of Practice.* 2nd edition. McGraw-Hill Book Co., New York.

Pearson, A. 1983. Primary nursing. *Nursing Times.* 5 October, pp.37–8.

Pearson, A. (ed) 1987. *Nursing Quality Measurement. Quality Assurance Methods for Peer Review.* HM+M Nursing Publications, John Wiley and Sons, London.

Phaneuf, M. C. 1972. *The Nursing Audit, Profile for Excellence.* Appleton-Century-Crofts, New York.

Rogers, C. R. 1961. *On Becoming a Person.* Houghton Mifflin Co., Boston.

Roper, N., Logan, W. W. and Tierney, A. J. 1981. *Learning to Use the Process of Nursing.* Churchill Livingstone, Edinburgh.

Roper, N., Logan, W. W. and Tierney, A. J. (Eds) 1983a. *Using a Model for Nursing.* Churchill Livingstone, Edinburgh.

Roper, N., Logan, W. W. and Tierney, A. J. 1983b. A model for nursing. *Nursing Times.* 2 March, pp.24–7.

Roper, N., Logan, W. W. and Tierney, A. J. 1985. *The Elements of Nursing.* 2nd edition. Churchill Livingstone, Edinburgh.

Salvage, J. 1985. *The Politics of Nursing.* Heinemann, London.

Slater, D. 1967. *The Slater Nursing Competencies Scale.* Wayne State University, Detroit.

Sundeen, S. J., Stuart, G. W., Rankin, E. and Cohen, S. A. 1981. *Nurse-Client Interaction.* C. V. Mosby Co., St Louis.

Tutton, L. 1987. My very own nurse. *Nursing Times.* 23 September, pp.27–9.

Ujhely, G. B. 1968. *Determinants of the Nurse-Patient Relationship.* Springer Publishing Co. Inc., New York.

Wandelt, M. and Ager, J. 1974. *Quality Patient Care Scale.* Appleton-Century-Crofts, New York.

Williams, K. 1974. Ideologies of nursing – their meanings and implications. *Nursing Times.* Occasional Paper, 8 August, p.8.

Wright, D. 1984. An introduction to the evaluation of nursing care: a review of the literature. *Journal of Advanced Nursing*, 9, pp.457–67.

Wright, S. 1987. Patient centred practice. *Nursing Times.* 23 September, pp.24–7.

Yura, H. and Walsh, M. B. 1978. *The Nursing Process.* 3rd edition. Appleton-Century-Crofts, New York.

HEALTH AND ILLNESS

CONTENTS

▶ **The meaning of health** 41
Maintaining health – whose responsibility? 43
Economic and social factors affecting health 44

▶ **Becoming ill** 45
Health needs and the provision of health care 46
Becoming a patient 47

▶ **Prevention of ill health** 47
Primary prevention 48
Secondary prevention 48
Tertiary prevention 48

▶ **Nurses as health educators** 49

▶ **Nurses as role models for healthy living** 51

▶ **Further study** 52

▶ **References** 52

Two of the competencies of a nurse are to:

advise on the promotion of health and prevention of illness

recognize situations that may be detrimental to the health and well-being of the individual

A nurse whose practice reflects these competencies will, hopefully, be someone who enables people to develop their knowledge about the principles of healthy living and their awareness of the health choices that they can make by means of evaluating the known risks to health of certain components of life-style. The nurse will also be on hand to give support to people whilst they cope with and adapt to their changed life-style.

Nurses can help patients achieve these changes by setting aside specific time to teach patients and their relatives, but, and perhaps more realistically, the nurse will also need to take up actively opportunities to discuss and inform about health choices as and when they occur in everyday nursing contacts with people.

This chapter will introduce you to some of the dimensions of the concept of health and serve as a starting point from which you can develop your awareness of this fundamental subject area in nursing.

From this starting point you can think about the beliefs and values you hold about being healthy and evaluate how they are reflected in your life-style. This chapter goes on to discuss issues such as personal responsibility for health, and the contribution to health made by society's provision of services. The prevention of ill health and the role of nurses as health educators and role models for healthy life-styles is also outlined.

THE MEANING OF HEALTH

What does being healthy mean to you?

Take a piece of paper and write down ten ideas you have about what being healthy means for you.

Get a friend to do the same thing and compare your lists.

Try to put your ideas about being healthy into some sort of ranking order – from those of the most importance to those of least importance.

Try to categorize your ideas and to determine whether they relate to your physical, emotional or spiritual health.

Other similar activities you may like to try can be found in Elwes and Simnett (1985).

During your reflections you may have also recalled past situations when doing the same exercise would have produced a different sort of list. For example, after fracturing a leg you would have been frustrated and concerned about your lack of mobility and might have been preoccupied with your physical health. Alternatively, after having a viral illness you may have been left depressed and tired and this would have made you concerned about your emotional as well as your physical health.

People attach personal meanings to such ideas as being healthy, being fit, being unwell and being ill. Consider, for instance, the definitions of health given in the opening chapters of DHSS 1980, Coutts and Hardy 1985 and Elwes and Simnett 1985.

Individuals have personal and subjective meanings for health which may contrast with those developed by 'experts'. One definition that is often reproduced is that of the World Health Organization (1947), where health is held to be:

> a state of complete physical, mental and social well-being, rather than solely as an absence of disease.

Elwes and Simnett (1985) identify a number of dimensions to the concept of health – that of physical, mental, emotional, social, spiritual and societal health. Coutts and Hardy (1985) remind us that health is not a static state of affairs, such as the WHO definition might lead us to believe, but rather a dynamic and changing state of affairs. Some people may feel 'unhealthy' at different times in their lives following specific events. In addition to our examples of a leg fracture or recovery from a viral infection, we can usefully include being bereaved or becoming unemployed. But equally well others may not see themselves as being unhealthy at those times.

The Open University (1985) see health as being related to the interactions of three factors during a person's lifetime:

1 his biological state;
2 his personal history and passage through life events such as puberty, marriage and retirement;
3 the society in which he lives – its economy and the way in which it provides health care.

Furthermore, these three factors need to be considered within the perspective of history, with its consequent changing expectations and definitions of health.

Elwes and Simnett (1985) distinguish between mental health,

emotional health, social health and spiritual health. These four dimensions encompass the abilities of people:

— to think clearly and coherently; to recognize emotions such as fear, joy, grief and anger and to express such emotions appropriately
— to cope with stress, tension, depression and anxiety
— to have the ability to make and maintain relationships with other people
— to have ways of achieving peace of mind

Are you surprised by the Elwes and Simnett definition relating to mental health?

Does it fit in with your picture of mental illness as an absence of mental health?

MAINTAINING HEALTH – WHOSE RESPONSIBILITY?

Some authors argue that the provision of health care services to cure illness have less of an impact on people's health than society's provision of a living environment which fosters the conditions for health in the first place. Consider the arguments put forward by Illich 1975, McKeown 1976, DHSS 1980 and Health Education Council 1987.

It can be argued that it is a personal responsibility to maintain one's own health by looking after oneself and by seeking out help and advice for health problems when they arise.

Another view takes into account that we also need to live in a healthy society and environment because this will closely affect our personal health. This view maintains that society provides, by means of local and central government agencies, services which enable individuals to be healthy. The provision of drinkable water, sewerage systems, legislation to ensure the provision of wholesome food and clean air are examples. They have a great impact on any individual's ability to be healthy. The provision of satisfactory housing, employment, income and education will also affect an individual's health, and again these aspects are not entirely controlled by individuals acting on their own.

For example, being able to cope with and gain satisfaction from your job is likely to be an important factor in maintaining your personal health. If health problems intervene and affect your performance this will be of great importance to you. Equally, if you do not have a job this may affect your health and give rise to physical and emotional ill health.

Opinions vary about the effects of unemployment on health. What do you think? For useful references, see Norman 1984, Laurance 1986, Wagstaff 1986 and Arber 1987.

ECONOMIC AND SOCIAL FACTORS AFFECTING HEALTH

So far we have touched on the way in which the concept of health is defined, and we have acknowledged the subjective nature of the definitions given by individuals. Our health is partly determined by choices we make about our individual life-styles and partly by the circumstances in which we live, particularly those which enable us to be free to make such choices.

It would appear that our chances of good health and long life can be calculated or predicted to some extent. The Black Report (DHSS 1980) drew attention to the relative inequalities in health between social classes. There are problems in defining to everyone's satisfaction what social class means and that is acknowledged in the Report. The definition used is:

> segments of the population sharing broadly similar types and levels of resources, with broadly similar styles of living and (for some sociologists) some shared perception of their collective condition.
>
> (DHSS 1980, p.13)

Social classes are listed in the Report in this way:

Social class 1	Professional e.g. accountant, doctor, lawyer
Social class 2	Intermediate e.g. manager, schoolteacher, nurse
Social class 3n	Skilled non-manual; e.g. clerical worker, secretary, shop assistant
Social class 3m	Skilled manual, e.g. bus driver, butcher, coal-face worker, carpenter
Social class 4	Partly skilled e.g. agricultural worker, bus conductor, postman
Social class 5	Unskilled e.g. labourer, cleaner, dock worker

The working party which produced the Report concluded that there were marked inequalities in health between the social classes. They used mortality rates (death rates) for the different social classes as evidence for this. For example, at birth and in the first month of life twice as many babies of parents in social class 5 die, as those from parents in social class 1.

The Report shows evidence that personal reporting of 'long-standing illness' were twice as high for the unskilled manual male workers and two and a half times as high for unskilled manual female workers as males and females respectively in the professional classes.

Obtain a copy of the Report in its original form or in its easily available paperback version (Townsend and Davidson, 1982) and consider its findings and recommendations.

More recent evidence to support the findings of the Black Report about inequalities in health between the social classes has been reported (H.E.C. 1987). However, the use of death rates in the age group

15–64 as evidence of 'inequalities in health' has been questioned (Illesley and Le Grand 1987).

BECOMING ILL

Health, as we have seen, is defined subjectively and therefore differently by individual persons. Being healthy relates to our well-being emotionally and socially and not just physically. At some point though we may feel ourselves to be healthy no longer, but ill, and in need of 'expert' help in order to put things right.

It is thought that people who come forward to attend a doctor's surgery are the tip of the 'clinical iceberg' of ill health in society. In other words people may develop niggling pains and notice changes in their bodies but will explain them away and not see themselves as being ill. They may see such pains and changes as being normal – due to age, some activity they have or have not done, something they have eaten. They may alter their behaviour to accommodate the problem by going to bed earlier, by 'slowing down' and resting more, by avoiding suspect foods or by taking a day off from work.

At a later stage people may decide that the problem is no longer 'normal' or 'liveable with' and it is at this point that they may consult with others, particularly those thought to have some understanding about illness such as knowledgeable neighbours, the chemist, a person who trained as a nurse. If these people are not able to help, eventually they do go and see the doctor.

Armstrong (1980) suggests that there are 'triggers' which send people to their doctor's surgery. Some of these 'social triggers' are:

1 interference with work or physical activity;
2 the occurrence of an interpersonal crisis, perhaps a change in relationships, which prevents the person from coping with and tolerating the symptom;
3 interference with social or personal relationships;
4 passing a deadline set by the person by which time the symptom should have gone away;
5 pressure on the person from other people that he should consult a doctor.

Bear these possible 'triggers' in mind when you listen to people explaining why they visited their GP or the Accident and Emergency Department of your hospital. (And see also Jocelyn Cornwell's book, 1984, with its accounts by people from London's East End of their health and health problems.)

Reflect back to when you last decided to consult a doctor about a health problem. Try answering these questions:

When had you noticed the problem?

How did you explain its significance to yourself?

Did you share your concern with other people?

When you decided to go to see a doctor – what was the deciding factor for you?

What label or medical diagnosis were you given for your problem?

HEALTH NEEDS AND THE PROVISION OF HEALTH CARE

Armstrong (1980) suggests that a person's use of the health services which are provided depends on three factors:

1   their actual need for the services provided;
2   their 'illness behaviour', i.e. what they do when they feel that they are 'ill';
3   the availability of health services.

He discusses two influential analyses that have been put forward to explain people's use of health services.

THE 'INVERSE CARE LAW' (Tudor Hart 1971)

This proposes that people with the greatest need for health services have the poorest provision of them, and those with the least need have the best services.

DOCTOR-INDUCED DISEASE – IATROGENESIS (Illich 1975)

This viewpoint maintains that for the ill person the very use of doctors and the treatments they recommend produce further ill health for the person concerned. In other words, the treatment may produce further illness. In addition, Illich argues that people have become over-dependent on the so-called 'experts' in health care and this over-dependence produces further apparent need for doctors and sophisticated treatments and results in people believing and feeling that they need more of both.

Try to investigate these two issues further and produce a written account of the position you would take to argue that:

People with the greatest health-care needs get the poorest provision of health-care services and this is unjust.

'High tech' medicine produces more problems than solutions.

BECOMING A PATIENT

Talcott Parsons, a sociologist (1951), has described what he saw as the expectations held within Western society about becoming a 'patient'. He proposed that there are two privileges and two obligations that come with becoming a patient.

The 'privileges' are that the patient is excused the obligations of his or her usual role. First, a person is not expected to go to work, and is excused some of the normal social obligations such as being nice to people and joining in social activities. Second, in Western society a patient is not usually held to be responsible for his illness.

The obligations are that the person must want to get better, and must co-operate with the treatment and with the doctor.

Are people held to be responsible for their illnesses?

Reflect back on the attitudes that are displayed about:

1   people with AIDS;
2   people who become severely injured following a road traffic accident when it is known that they had been drinking alcohol;
3   women who develop cancer of the cervix;
4   people who have been smokers who develop cancer of the lung.

Patients have their health problem assessed by a doctor and a descriptive label is given to it – the medical diagnosis. (For a further discussion about 'labelling' and the controversies surrounding the diagnosis of mental illness see Clare 1976 and Szasz 1972.)

Some of these labels or medical diagnoses become themselves another problem for a patient. Consider the problems which may arise for the following:

a person with a diagnosis of cancer;

a person with a diagnosis of a 'mental illness' such as schizophrenia.

PREVENTION OF ILL HEALTH

In reading about the prevention of ill health in the health education literature you will come across the following concepts:

> the primary prevention of ill health
> the secondary prevention of ill health
> the tertiary prevention of ill health

This is a summary of what these concepts mean.

PRIMARY PREVENTION

This centres around activities designed to try to prevent illness occurring in the first place. For example, if ill health can be linked to behaviour an attempt can be made to try to help people realize the implications of their behaviour and its relationship to the probability of their developing illness at some time in the future. This may then motivate them to change their behaviour.

An example is that of the health education programmes which aim to stop children and young people from taking up the habit of smoking. The intention behind this is to prevent them developing the diseases which are linked with smoking – coronary heart disease, diseases of the circulatory system, cancer of the lungs and bronchus, and chronic bronchitis and emphysema.

Health education in schools

Were you exposed to health education whilst at school?

What was taught?

Who did the teaching?

What form did the teaching take?

Was it effective for you?

Other examples of primary prevention are fluoridation of the water supply, teaching dental hygiene to young people to prevent dental caries and gum disease, and immunization of babies and young children against the potentially fatal childhood diseases of diphtheria, whooping cough and polio.

SECONDARY PREVENTION

These include activities designed to detect and treat early manifestations of disease by screening people who by and large consider themselves healthy. An example would be taking blood pressure recordings of all people attending a general practice in order to detect hypertension. Other examples include the provision of screening facilities for the detection of breast and cervical cancer.

TERTIARY PREVENTION

This is reflected in efforts directed towards preventing the potential complications of established illness and minimizing the limitations on a person's life-style. Some examples of tertiary prevention include teaching and advising people with diabetes mellitus, a stoma or a myocardial infection how to care for themselves and maintain their health and well-being. In all these examples the intention is to help people live a full life again.

Devise a list of as many occupational roles of nurses as you can think of (e.g. hospital nurse, school nurse) and then outline how they may be involved in the primary, secondary and tertiary prevention of ill health in the populations they serve.

NURSES AS HEALTH EDUCATORS

One of the competencies of a nurse, as outlined at the beginning of this chapter, is that of being able to give advice to people about health and the prevention of illness. In this advisory capacity the nurse takes on the role of a health educator.

Coutts and Hardy (1985) explore different models of health education. They consider that nurses, in taking on the task of health education and patient teaching, usually subscribe to the model of health education which is an educational one. In other words the way to influence a person's ability to make choices about health is a matter of educating them first.

Reflect back over your last time on duty.

1   Do you feel you assisted a patient in any way to develop their awareness of the health choices open to them?

2   Do you recall a specific situation in which you actively and deliberately set about teaching and advising a patient in relation to the primary, secondary and the tertiary prevention of ill health.

If you consider you did not do **1** or **2**, can you pinpoint a reason why not? What prevented you?

Some typical opportunities for health teaching may include: explanations to patients about forthcoming investigations, surgery and treatments; helping patients to understand how constipation can be prevented by eating food with a high fibre content and drinking fluids, and helping patients to maintain muscle tone by exercise even when confined to bed by teaching them and positively reinforcing their practice.

Wilson-Barnett (1983) offers many ideas about teaching patients who, for instance

— are diabetic
— have stomas;
— have had a stroke;
— have psychiatric disorders;
— are incontinent;
— have had heart problems;
— are recovering from surgery.

Some of the key points to consider when teaching patients are:

1   To plan your teaching after taking into consideration what the patient needs to know and what he or she knows to start with.

2   To consider how many teaching sessions will be needed, what is to be taught in each, and how the key points will be communicated to the person learning.

3   To choose the 'right' *time* to teach, when the person is ready and shows an interest in the subject matter and feels that they have a need to learn.

4   To choose the 'right' *place* to teach, where you will not be interrupted and it is quiet.

5   To use a number of ways of stimulating learning by getting the person actively involved. Use as many senses as possible by touching equipment, looking, listening and talking about the points to be understood and remembered.

6   To enable the person to practise a manual skill, such as giving themselves an injection, by setting aside opportunities to practise by themselves and under your supervision.

7   To emphasize the key points by repeating the information and inviting the person to ask questions, and by providing them with a written record or set of instructions about the topic learned.

You may have also found yourself as a nurse really wanting to help patients to maintain and develop their health, not just to deal with their ill health, and this is a difficult undertaking. You may be unwilling to give advice to others when either you do not believe it sufficiently yourself because you have not incorporated it into your own life-style, or you may suspect that any advice you give is at best partial and may itself be the subject of controversy and alternative viewpoints by 'experts' in the field.

You may find it uncomfortable to discuss some matters – healthy eating, smoking and taking exercise, for example – if you already feel somewhat guilty about your own habits. A potential solution may be to consider again the literature about a healthy life-style which is widely available in libraries, bookshops and from established sources such as the Health Education Authority. The Open University/Health Education Council (1980) pack 'Health Choices' may be useful. A summary of the healthy living practices that it explores is outlined below. It is suggested by the team who devised the pack that each person appraise the topics for themselves.

—   Reassessing health for oneself and making decisions to change or not
—   Reconsidering personal relationships and deciding whether change is required
—   Reconsidering fitness and whether change is needed
—   Reconsidering eating habits
—   Reconsidering smoking/drinking/drug taking habits
—   Considering stress and its management

— Considering other states of being, such as anxiety and depression
— Reconsidering one's sex life

Obtain a package from the Health Education Authority about smoking, and in particular focus on the booklet aimed at nurses.

Take note of the suggestions given about helping patients to decide to stop smoking. Start to develop your own knowledge about the effects of smoking and useful practical strategies that can be shared with and explored by patients about giving up the habit.

Nurses can feel that the evidence about the effects of smoking on health are convincing. However, you may find that such 'incontrovertible' evidence is not available for such topics as nutrition and exercise, for example. How will you deal with these topics where medical and scientific evidence is lacking or apparently contradictory, when responding to patients' requests for information and advice?

NURSES AS ROLE MODELS FOR HEALTHY LIVING

Our attitudes and behaviour are influenced by the direct and indirect influence of other people. People can actively behave in certain ways in order to influence us, as parents do with their children, for example. On the other hand, people may not intend to influence our behaviour but do so unintentionally. This type of social influence on behaviour is called modelling. (See Baron and Byrne 1981, ch.6; and Coutts and Hardy 1985, pp.82–101.)

This concept of modelling or observational learning is held to be an important process in influencing attitudes. Psychologists have observed that in situations where people say one thing but with their behaviour demonstrate another viewpoint, it is their behaviour that is the factor that influences other people by means of modelling.

Consider this statement made in the Health Education Council's booklet, 'Helping people to stop smoking. A guide for hospital nurses', on page 2:

As a hospital nurse you provide a 'role model' – someone who sets an example by their own behaviour – for the patient. In a recent study, only 18 per cent of patients said they would accept a nurse's advice about smoking if they knew she smoked.

Do you think it is fair to nurses to expect them to be role models of healthy living practices, as is implied in the H.E.C.'s booklet?

It may be that you view yourself as a health educator who, by means of listening and talking with patients, enables them, if they want to, to choose to make changes in their life-styles. Here again, good communication skills are vital because it is more a matter of the nurse being a 'listening ear' and a 'sounding board' for a patient, whilst he or she grapples with making decisions about life-style, rather than an instructor of 'what to do' to be more healthy.

One of the fundamental principles in moral philosophy is that of respect for persons. This, in terms of health education, brings with it as a consequence an acceptance of the autonomy of individuals and their rights to make choices.

Do you feel that knowledge and acceptance of the above principle will help you in your dealings with patients who do not want to make health choices in the 'desired' direction?

FURTHER STUDY

1   As part of the nursing care of patients you may find it useful to use health education materials produced by the Health Education Authority or by your own Health Authority.
(*a*)   Visit your local Health Education Authority offices and critically examine the educational materials they have.
(*b*)   Choose a current health education campaign, for example that associated with AIDS, and assess its usefulness and limitations.
(*c*)   Consider patient information material produced in your Health Authority. Are there any omissions in the range of material produced? Have you any proposals, or indeed can you assist in remedying the omissions?

2   Check in your library for articles about health, health education and nurses as health educators.

3   Examine the 'strategic plan' of your health district for background information about the allocation of resources to the area of health education and promotion.

4   Liaise with your teacher in organizing a health education officer to speak to your student group about local initiatives being undertaken in health education and promotion in your area.

REFERENCES

Arber, S. 1987. Social class, non-employment and chronic illness: continuing the inequalities in health debate. *British Medical Journal*, 294, 25 April, pp.1069–73.

Armstrong, D. 1980. *An Outline of Sociology as Applied to Medicine*. John Wright and Sons Ltd, Bristol.

Baron, R. A. and Byrne, D. 1981. *Social Psychology: Understanding Human Interaction*. 3rd edition., Allyn and Bacon Inc, New York.

Clare, A. 1976. *Psychiatry in Dissent*. Tavistock Publications, London.

Cornwell, J. 1984. *Hard-earned Lives. Accounts of Health and Illness from East London.* Tavistock Publications, London.

Coutts, L. C. and Hardy, L. K. 1985. *Teaching for Health. The Nurse as Health Educator.* Churchill Livingstone, Edinburgh.

D.H.S.S. 1980. *Inequalities in Health. (The Black Report)* HMSO, London.

Elwes, L. and Simnet, J. 1985. *Promoting Health. A Practical Guide to Health Education.* John Wiley and Sons, London.

Health Education Council, 1987. *The Health Divide: Inequalities in Health in the 1980s.* Health Education Council, London.

Illesley, R. and Le Grand, J. 1987. *Measuirement of Inequality.* Discussion paper No. 12. The Welfare State Programme. Suntory–Toyota International Centre for Economics and Related Disciplines, London School of Economics.

Illich, I. 1975. *Medical Nemesis.* Calder and Boyars, London.

Laurance, J. 1986. Unemployment: health hazards. *New Society*, 75, 21 March, pp.492–3.

McKeown, T. 1976. *The Role of Medicine: Dream, Mirage or Nemesis?* The Nuffield Provincial Hospital Trust, London.

Norman, A. 1984. Out of work – out of health. *Nursing Mirror*, 11 April, p.16.

Open University, Health Education Council and Scottish Health Education Unit. 1980. *The Good Health Guide.* Harper and Row, London.

Open University, 1985. *Birth to Old Age. Health in Transition.* Open University, Milton Keynes.

Parsons, T. 1951. *The Social System.* The Free Press of Glencoe, New York.

Szasz, T. S. 1972. *The Myth of Mental Illness.* Paladin, London.

Townsend, P. and Davidson, N. 1982. *Inequalities in Health. The Black Report.* Penguin, London.

Tudor Hart, J. 1971. The inverse care law. *Lancet*, 1, pp.405–12.

Wagstaff, A. 1986. Unemployment and health: some pitfalls for the unwary. *Health Trends.* November, 4.18, pp.79–81.

Wilson-Barnett, J. (ed) 1983. *Patient Teaching.* Churchill Livingstone, Edinburgh.

World Health Organization. 1947. *Constitution of the WHO.* Chronicle of the WHO, 1.3, p.1.

THE USE OF RESEARCH IN NURSING

CONTENTS

▶ **The history of research in nursing** 59
The effect of early research on the profession 59
The relevance of nursing research today 60
Stages of research 61

▶ **The research process** 62
Stage 1: Identifying the problem 63
Stage 2: Collecting essential facts 63
Stage 3: Selecting an hypothesis 63
Stages 4 & 5: Selecting a suitable design and collecting essential data 65
Stage 6: Analysing and evaluating the data 69
Stage 7: Reporting the research and its findings 73
Research funding 74
The ethical dimensions of a research project 75

▶ **Reading a research report** 75
Some initial critical questions 76
More detailed questions 76

▶ **Further study** 78

▶ **References** 78

The United Kingdom Central Council for Nurses, Health Visitors and Midwives (1986) suggests that one of the key competencies of a nurse is the ability to:

> demonstrate an appreciation of research and use relevant literature and research as an aid to nursing practice.

Make a list of the many irregularities contained within this spoof study and the way in which it is presented.

THE MOST SUITABLE THING TO WEAR?

It has recently come to my notice, and that of my colleagues, that there is dissension within the profession about the most suitable attire for nurses to wear working in the wards.

Most of us agree now that the traditional full skirts, starched collars and decorative?! caps are outdated and impractical.

The following piece of research, therefore, was carried out to prove this very point.

I decided, for the sake of comparison, to confine my study to one aspect of a nurse's daily work – that is lifting. A sample of nurses was selected randomly, half of whom wore trousers, half of whom wore traditional nurses' dresses. Obviously, economic constraints made it impossible to buy new trousers for nurses, so for this reason I compared lifting practices between male and female nurses.

Obviously, too, I had to ensure that all nurses had been taught the same lifting techniques, so I confined my study to 30 student nurses who had been taught initially by the same teacher in the School of Nursing.

My sample consisted of 15 male and 15 female students. I watched each of them lift 3 times and noted if they were good or bad lifts. I also monitored their work area.

I arrived at the following significant results.

WORK AREA

Subject		General Medical ward	General Surgical ward	Care of the elderly unit	Paediatrics
MALE (Trouser Wearing)	1		✓✓X		
	2	✓✓			
	3				✓✓✓
	4				✓✓✓
	5			XX✓	
	6				✓✓✓
	7		X✓✓		
	8	✓X✓			
	9		✓✓✓		
	10				✓✓✓
	11				✓✓✓
	12			XX✓	
	13		✓✓✓		
	14	✓✓X			
	15				✓✓✓
FEMALE (Dress Wearing)	16			XXX	
	17	XX✓			
	18		✓X✓		
	19			XXX	
	20	X✓X			
	21		X✓✓		
	22			X✓X	
	23	XXX			
	24		XX✓		
	25				✓✓✓
	26			✓XX	
	27	X✓X			
	28		✓XX		
	29			XX✓	
	30				✓✓✓

✓ = Good Lift
X = Bad Lift

It will be clearly seen from the above tables that $\frac{36}{45}$ lifts by trouser wearing students were good, whereas only $\frac{17}{45}$ lifts by dress wearing students were good.

The hypothesis, therefore, is clearly proven.

The aims of this chapter are to give you some understanding of the importance of nursing research to the profession, and to enable you to read reports with critical appreciation.

THE HISTORY OF RESEARCH IN NURSING

THE EFFECT OF EARLY RESEARCH UPON THE PROFESSION

In the long history of nursing, it is probably true to say that the importance of research has only recently been recognized by the profession as a whole.

Nursing has, for many years, been considered a practical profession and, historically, more emphasis has been placed on the 'doing' than the 'thinking'. This may be because the early apprenticeship system, which commanded obedience rather than questioning, founded an ethos by which nurses traditionally tended to accept ideas and knowledge from outside authorities, or it may be because the general low status of women had hitherto hindered the lack of an enquiring approach to nursing. Whatever the reason, development of the partnership between practitioner and investigator has, perhaps, been rather slow to emerge. Yet, if the ultimate goal of improved patient care is to be achieved, this is a partnership which must develop.

Today's nurses cannot claim to be the first to appreciate the importance of research awareness. Individual nurses in the past have addressed the need to base policy and practice on the findings of investigative studies. For instance, Florence Nightingale, a member of the Statistical Society, presented a paper entitled 'Uniform Hospital Policy'. The information for her survey was gathered from hospitals all over Europe. This, in view of the fact that the paper was compiled without secretarial help and written by hand, was a remarkable feat. Equally remarkable is the fact that Miss Nightingale managed to write a 1,000 page report for the Commission on the Crimean War.

Although these studies established the importance of gathering facts and information as a basis for change or reformation, the relevance of nursing research was not to be universally appreciated at that time.

Research studies were, however, carried out at the turn of the century and nurse education provided a forum for investigation, particularly in America where, apparently, there was more awareness of the need for systematic study of nursing practice and the teaching of nursing than there was in Great Britain.

During the late 1950s and 1960s, however, nurses in this country began to carry out research, an example of this being the studies undertaken by Doreen Norton (1957) in her work with the elderly and their care.

Her work precipitated the manufacture of purpose-built chairs with high seats and the use of raised seats and hand rails in toilets – equipment that today we take for granted. You may be familiar with the Norton Score – a Pressure Points Scale devised by Doreen Norton as a result of her work with the elderly. (If you are using the Norton Scale to assess young patient's liability to developing pressure sores . . . think! Is this appropriate?) The profound effect of Norton's work on nursing practice, then, is an illustration of the relevance of nursing research.

Scientific research has been responsible for most of the major advances made by our society in the last century, yet nursing has relied heavily upon 'folk lore' and 'word of mouth' information. Indeed, as recently as 1969, Virginia Henderson felt bound to state that: 'Most aspects of basic nursing, including the nurse's approach to the patient, are steeped in tradition and passed from one generation of nurses to another. Too often they are routine without rhyme or reason. They are learned by imitation and taught with little if any reference to the underlying sciences.'

Nursing has also borrowed facts from other sciences without necessarily testing them scientifically to determine how well they might serve in their new role. A graphic example of this 'folk lore' has been the practice of applying egg white and oxygen to pressure sores, and many nurses of the generation who used this treatment would possibly state very firmly that this was an effective method of promoting healing and that the egg white was a good source of protein which encouraged the process. Here, then, information was 'borrowed' from other sciences and 'used' by nurses.

Norton's research of the 1950s and 1960s suggests that relief of the pressure is the most effective way of healing sores and now, with the benefit of hindsight, we can conclude that it was probably the very movement of patients in order to apply the oxygen for periods of time which was fundamental to the improvement in the skin condition.

Are you now carrying out any procedures which you feel may not be based upon sound reasoning or nursing investigation? Think about this, as you may find a use for your idea later on in this chapter.

THE RELEVANCE OF NURSING RESEARCH TODAY

Current research, then, is a tool which nurses can employ in studying their practice to obtain the scientific evidence for validating that practice. The findings of their investigations should be used by them in their future work.

Nurses can participate in research in several ways. They might observe nursing care, the response of patients to that care, and then raise questions which may require further study.

One example of such a study was carried out by Iles and Newman (1975), who were nurses at the London Hospital. They observed nurses caring for patients who were receiving intravenous therapy, and their exploratory study highlighted the difficulties and the number of interruptions which nurses experience whilst administering care relating to the infusions. They published their findings to bring them to the attention of colleagues within the profession.

A second way of participating in nursing research is to assist in the collection of information and facts (data) for a research project and, of course, a principle way would be to run a study yourself.

Strictly speaking, nursing research is concerned with the systematic investigation of nursing practice itself and of the effect of this practice on patient care or individual, family or community health. However, the general term 'nursing research' often refers to research into nurse education and nursing administration.

The purpose of research is to provide new knowledge by finding valid answers to questions that have been raised, or valid solutions to problems that have been indentified. Unlike problem solving, the problem selected for research is not related to a particular patient or to an immediate concern, but to the care of patients generally, or to a specific group of patients.

STAGES OF RESEARCH

In simple terms, scientific research involves the following stages:

1 **Identifying the problem** and delineating it clearly so that it becomes a manageable research question.
2 **Collecting essential facts** pertaining to the problem, e.g. reviewing the literature, selecting relevant theories which might help to explain the problem.
3 **Selecting an hypothesis** – this will be discussed in more depth later in this chapter.
4 **Setting up a suitable design** or method for the study.
5 **Collecting the essential data** required for evaluating the hypothesis.
6 **Analysing and evaluating the data** in terms of the hypothesis.
7 **Reporting the research and its findings.**

If the research process is totally new to you, then you will probably not yet clearly understand all of the above stages. It is hoped, however, that by the end of this chapter you will have gained more insight into the process.

Nursing research is of relevance today in several ways:

1 It may be used to study the various aspects of a specific problem of care.
2 It may be used to compare two or more methods of care.
3 It can be used to evaluate the use of a specific approach to care. This usually involves comparing the approach of one group to that of a control group.
4 It is used to evaluate a model of nursing.

One way of gaining information about ongoing or completed research is to consult the quarterly publication produced by the Index of Nursing Research at the DHSS called *Nursing Research Abstracts*. If you can obtain a copy, choose a topic which interests you and check the Index to see if there is any ongoing or recently completed research in this area.

It is also fascinating to obtain back copies of this journal so that you can identify areas of importance in the nursing profession throughout the last decade. Certainly, the 1970s produced a wealth of research literature.

As an exercise, see if you can find a reference to Jill Macleod Clark's research work on communication in nursing.

When did she do this?

How did she set about it?

As a direct result of Dr Macleod Clark's work, members of the nursing profession throughout the United Kingdom started to consider what they said to patients, what they did not say, how patients saw them and how they (the nurses) could become more astute about picking up patients non-verbal cues.

The impact on nurse education throughout the country was tremendous and the *Nursing Times* (1981) ran a series of articles relating to communication skills, having declared 1981 as the 'year of communication'.

See if you can find some *Nursing Times* articles for that series. You may find it useful reference for future chapters in this study aid.

THE RESEARCH PROCESS

It was suggested on page 60 that you should try to identify an area of nursing practice which you think requires systematic investigation. If you cannot think of one, perhaps there is an area of nurse education or administration which interests you.

Think of something which is not too complex, so that you can subject it, step by step, to a systematic process of investigation.

For the purposes of illustration, I shall refer back to the erstwhile common practice of treating pressure sores with egg-white and oxygen and apply the research stages to this as if I were, in fact, running a study to measure the effect of this practice in patient care.

Let us suppose that as a nurse some ten to fifteen years ago I had become aware in my own work area that the practice of applying egg-white and oxygen (O_2) to pressure sores was increasing, and that I wanted, in some way, to determine that this was an appropriate and effective form of nursing treatment.

STAGE 1: IDENTIFYING THE PROBLEM

The problem is that the practice of applying egg-white and O_2 seems to be increasing. I would like to have some research basis to support this practice if it is to continue.

Can you define the problem which you have identified for yourself? Having done so, what will your next steps be?

Until now I have only had an idea. I *think* I have identified a problem, but my observation is fairly subjective and could certainly not be used as a general statement about nursing practice everywhere! So perhaps my first step would be, on an informal basis, to contact nursing colleagues throughout the country to see whether this treatment is flourishing nationwide. If it appears that I have highlighted a national trend, then my next step would be to carry out a literature search.

STAGE 2: COLLECTING ESSENTIAL FACTS

In undertaking a literature search for my stated problem, I would search library catalogues for information/literature about:

> The properties of egg-white
> The properties of oxygen
> The healing process
> Pressure area care
> The treatment of pressure sores.

Have you thought of key topic areas which you may need to read about in order to research the problem which you have identified?

At this stage of the process, a potential researcher may realize that the stated problem has already been addressed in a previously published work. The dilemma then to be faced is:

Is there a case for replicating the earlier piece of work?

or

Is there another approach which could be used to research the same problem which may give support to conclusions already reached?

or

At this point, is it more sensible to abandon the idea altogether?

STAGE 3: SELECTING AN HYPOTHESIS

An hypothesis is:

—   a supposition
—   a proposition assured for the sake of argument
—   a theory to be proved or disproved by reference to the facts

— a professional explanation of anything (*Chambers 20th Century Dictionary*)

In other words, when formulating an hypothesis the researcher is making a supposition which scientific investigation may or may not support.

Can you formulate an hypothesis for researching the problem which you have identified?

If you have found this at all difficult, it may help you to break your thought processes down into three stages:

1   A declaration (e.g. 'I am going to describe the effect of egg-white and O_2 on pressure sores').
2   A question (e.g. 'Do egg-white and O_2 reduce the time which it takes for a pressure sore to heal?').
3   A hypothesis (e.g. that egg-white and O_2 reduce the healing time of pressure sores).

THE NULL HYPOTHESIS

At this stage I would like to suggest that a null hypothesis would be more approriate.

A null hypothesis is one which suggests that
'A' will not affect 'B'

The null hypothesis for my proposed experiment, then, would be that the use of egg-white and O_2 will have no effect on the healing rate of pressure sores.

Can you think of any advantages for using a null hypothesis rather than an hypothesis?

An hypothesis may suggest researcher bias. My proposed hypothesis suggests that I anticipate that egg-white and O_2 will treat pressure sores effectively, where as a null hypothesis is, perhaps, more indicative of an 'open-minded' approach to the experiment.

A null hypothesis also presents a sounder foundation for deductive reasoning: If an experiment does support the null hypothesis that 'A' has no effect on 'B', then there may be a case for exploring the effect of 'C' on 'B', then 'D' and so on.

An experiment based on an hypothesis, however, may leave unanswered questions. For instance, let us suppose that I carried out my proposed study using an hypothesis, and I concluded that the findings did, indeed, support the theory that application of egg-white and O_2 expedites pressure sore healing. Can I be sure that nothing else has in any way influenced my results (the age of the patients, the type of ward, for example)? The answer to this question would have to be 'no!'.

If, however, I use a null hypothesis and a significant trend emerges from my findings, I can then proceed to investigate this trend further, knowing that I have a sound basis for doing so.

STAGES 4 AND 5: SELECTING A SUITABLE DESIGN AND COLLECTING ESSENTIAL DATA

This is a crucial stage of the whole process, and before you consider suitable methods for researching *your* identified problem, it may be of help to consider the ways in which I could set up an experiment to test the null hypothesis that the use of egg-white and O_2 will have no effect on the healing rate of pressure sores.

First of all, I will need access to patients with pressure sores, and I will need a device for assessing how rapidly these are healing. This should not be too difficult as a pressure sore is something which can be seen and literally measured with a ruler. If I then say, for example, that I will observe and measure the healing rate of 100 pressure sores treated with oxygen and egg-white, will I actually be able to produce any written statement which could be considered valid?

N.B. *A valid piece of research is one in which the methodology actually does test the hypothesis stated.*

I clearly need to take the process one stage further, and consider using a control group of patients.

In any experiment, the control group is treated in the same way as the experimental group except for the one specific point which is being tested.

I am testing effectiveness of egg-white and oxygen on pressure sores. If I wish to measure this treatment against a control, then I need to have access to patients with pressure sores which are treated by positioning them in the same way and for the same length of time as those in the experimental group (Group A). The only difference would be that those in the control group (Group B) do not have egg-white and oxygen applied to their pressure sores. Indeed, for true uniformity of subjects, all the patients should, if possible, have sores which are of the same diameter and same width.

If I then compared the rate of patients in group A with those in group B, should I be able to test my null hypothesis?

Can you see any problems here? You have, perhaps, identified the possibility of there being too many variables between the two groups.

Variables are factors outside an experiment which may effect its validity. For this reason variable factors should be controlled as closely as possible.

What variable factors may affect the validity of this experiment?

Firstly, are the patients in each group of 'like' kind? My initial literature search should have highlighted the fact that people who are malnourished and/or elderly do not heal as readily as those who are young or well nourished. Should I then confine my experiment to patients within a certain age group? This may control one variable factor to some extent. Should I also, perhaps, confine my experiment to patients within a certain range of weight? But, then, what about the diet of patients, the amount of independent movement which each of them can achieve, their level of consciousness?

It would seem that the variables are endless, which indeed they are when carrying out experiments involving people. This is a problem which, obviously, many nurse researchers encounter.

To avoid this problem, I could, in my example, decide to use a random sample of patients.

A random sample of the population is one which is chosen purely by chance. There is no uniformity or pre-set criteria.

By choosing a random sample, it could be argued that there is an equal chance for each group to be affected by external variables. At least there will be no overt consistent variable which would heavily bias or 'skew' the results. (An extreme example of 'result skewing' would be to conduct a survey of religious beliefs using a population of people leaving a Roman Catholic Church on a Sunday morning.)

Let us now summarize my research proposal.

GROUP A	GROUP B
50 patients with pressure sores, of between 2 and 5 cm in diameter. (Random Sample) Patients will be positioned so that the sore area is kept free of pressure at all times.	50 patients with pressure sores of between 2 and 5 cm in diameter. (Random Sample) Patients will be positioned so that the sore area is kept free from pressure at all times.
Patients treated 4 hourly, by application of ½ teaspoon of egg-white to sore. This to be followed by a 20 min flow of O_2 (Mark 6 on flow meter) to the sore.	There will be no other treatment.
DIAMETER OF SORE TO BE MEASURED DAILY.	DIAMETER OF SORE TO BE MEASURED DAILY.

The instructions for the treatment of patients in the experimental group (Group A) have to be very specific so that there are no variables within the same group.

At this stage it might be advisable to run a pilot study.

A pilot study is a small-scale experiment which is run in the same manner as the intended full-scale experiment. Its purpose is to identify any problems, in advance, so that these may be controlled.

The pilot study may, for example, highlight logistic problems such as limited availability of suitable patients, the difficulty for one researcher to visit such a large number of patients on a daily basis. It may be that I would have to settle for a smaller sample of patients, or I could engage the services of research assistants over a wide geographical area to carry out this phase of data gathering on my behalf.

At this point, can you identify the possible pros and cons for conducting personal interviews or distributing questionnaires? These are some of the points which you may have considered.

QUESTIONNAIRE	INTERVIEWS
Can reach many people in a short space of time.	Can be very time consuming.
May be misunderstood by subjects.	Allow for clarification and questioning.
Not all recipients reply.	If subjects agree to be interviewed, it usually takes place.
Not all recipients reply sensibly.	'Flippant' replies can be elicited.
Non-verbal cues, reactions, e.g. anxiety, may be missed.	Non-verbal reactions may be noted.

There are three principal research strategies. Firstly, there is empirical research. Empirical research is that in which information is obtained in the 'field' and from the study of subjects.

There are three main types of empirical research:

1 **Descriptive research** by which the researcher writes a case study of observed happenings and conducts a survey by interview or questionnaire to describe a situation.
2 **Experimental research** in which actual occurrences are described, but the situation is somewhat manipulated by using an experimental and control group of subjects.
3 **Action research** is a design within which an attempt is made to address the identified problem in some way, and the outcome of this change is evaluated.

Can you suggest an application of each of these research designs to the problem which I have identified?
Which research design have I actually proposed using?

By proposing the use of an experimental and control group of subjects, I was advocating an **experimental research** design. Had I chosen descriptive design, I would have used the technique of observing pressure sore treatment, commissioning research assistants to observe pressure sore treatment, or sending out questionnaires to conduct a survey of techniques in treating pressure sores. An action research project would have been appropriate if a change in pressure sore treatment had been implemented and that change evaluated.

It can be seen, then, that empirical research is the design commonly used in the clinical setting.

There are two other research strategies which you should, perhaps, become aware of, these are **Historical Research** and **Philosophical Research**. Historical research is that in which documents and reports are analysed with the aim of drawing conclusions which may have relevance for nursing today.

Such a researcher could, for example, consider the history of nurse education, its relevance or influence in nursing practice and draw conclusions for current nurse educators. Philosophical research is an attempt to enhance knowledge through reason and logic.

Such a researcher may, for example, seek to analyse the ideologies underpinning nurse education. To do this she may use similar primary sources to those of an historical researcher, and she may seek statements of belief and ideology from individual schools and colleges of nursing.

In addition she will examine concepts, values and beliefs used in order to produce a comprehensive analysis.

STAGE 6: ANALYSING AND EVALUATING THE DATA

The purpose of carrying out a scientific investigation is to elicit facts, new knowledge, new understanding, and a crucial part of 'writing up' such a piece of work must therefore be the account of the outcome.

The key word, I would suggest, is *clarity* of information, and if diagrams, tables, or graphs aid this clarity then it is appropriate to use them.

Unless you are already a statistician, you may need to seek expert help in analysing the data that you have collected. Some tests for analysis would be more appropriate for one investigation than another, but it is not in the remit of this text to address all aspects of statistical methodology. If you are interested, you may enjoy reading *How to Lie with Statistics* by Darrell Huff (1975) or *Statistics Without Tears* by Derek Rowntree (1981), either of which should provide you with a painless introduction to the subject!

I recommend that you read one of the above books, particularly if you do not understand the following terms:

a table of results
A pie chart
A scatter diagram
A bar chart
A graph.

To return to the pressure sores experiment, the first stage of analysis and evaluation would be a detailed synopsis of the time taken for the patients' pressure sores to heal. In the interests of clarity I could translate my findings into tabular form.

I would need to show a comparison between the control group and the experimental group.

Table to show healing time of pressure sores for patients in control and experimental groups.

Time taken for sores to heal	Actual number of pressures sores which took this length of time to heal		Percentage of pressure sores which took this length of time to heal	
	Group A	Group B	Group A	Group B
Less than 1 week	2	2	4%	4%
1–2 weeks	1	2	2%	4%
2–3 weeks	5	4	10%	8%
3–4 weeks	10	9	20%	18%
4–5 weeks	12	15	24%	30%
5–6 weeks	9	7	18%	14%
6–7 weeks	7	8	14%	16%
7–8 weeks	3	–	6%	–
More than 8 weeks	1	3	2%	6%
	50	50	100%	100%

Having considered the time taken, I would then try to identify any trends and discuss these more fully (e.g. patients of certain ages in both subject groups tended to demonstrate delayed healing, and patients in both groups who were deemed to be underweight took longer to heal than those who were of average weight for their height).

If a very definite trend has emerged, I could identify this diagrammatically by using, for example, a *pie chart*, which is a useful device for demonstrating the proportions of a response. This does not show precise information but indicates a trend.

Proportion of patients whose pressure sores took more than six weeks to heal (all subjects)

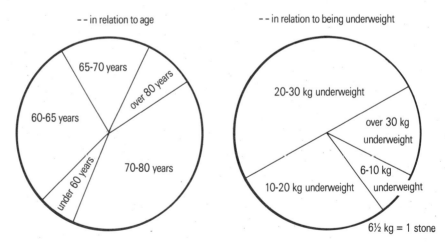

6½ kg = 1 stone

Another trend that I would almost certainly wish to explore would be that of the relationship between the initial size of the pressure sores and the time taken for them to heal. This could be simply represented on a scatter diagram.

Scatter diagram to show relationship between initial size of pressure sores and healing time

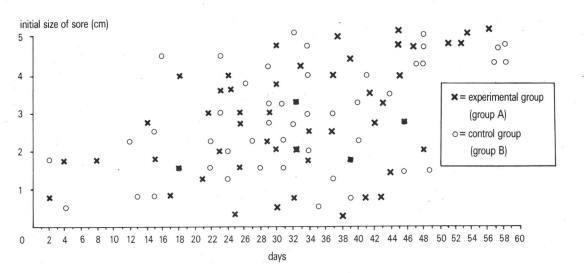

At this stage some conclusions will be drawn from the whole experiment, and the question to be asked is, did application of egg-white and O_2 significantly affect the healing rate of pressure sores?

A graph could be used here to illustrate the number of days it took for the sores of subjects in group A to heal in comparison with those of group B.

A graph to illustrate comparative healing time of pressure sores of patients in experimental group (A) and those in control group (B)

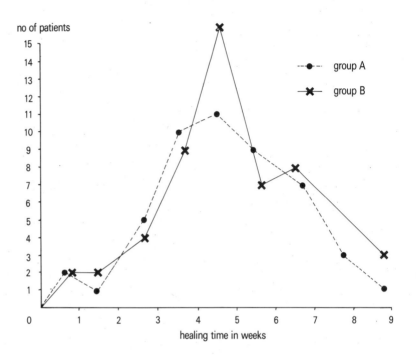

Alternatively, a bar chart could be used, although I would probably have to use two diagrams here, as to superimpose the results obtained from group A on to those of group B may result in a confusing chart.

Bar charts to illustrate the comparative healing time of pressure sores of patients in experimental group (A) and those in the control group (B)

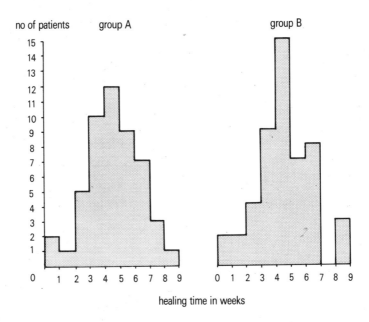

healing time in weeks

A word of caution about using graphs, charts, or any type of diagram! Do make sure that it is an accurate representation.

I am now ready to evaluate the methodology and results. Any faults in methodology (e.g. a bias of subjects) should be acknowledged.

STAGE 7: REPORTING THE RESEARCH AND ITS FINDINGS

This is a crucial stage, as it is here that the researcher considers whether the study has any implications for future health care. (Again I refer you to the implications of Jill Macleod Clark's study of nurses communication skills, page 62).

In writing up a piece of research, you will aid clarity if you open with an abstract, or synopsis, of the research problem design and its conclusions. This 'sets the scene'.

The report could then be set out, perhaps, in the following way:

Statement of the problem/hypothesis.
Discussion of the literature and observations which have precipitated this study.
Descriptions and explanations of the methodology.
Summary of the results.
Discussion of the possible implications of the research findings.
Conclusion.

Can you speculate on the conclusions which could emerge from your research proposal?

Do you envisage that your hypothesis/null hypothesis would be supported?

What would you infer, do you think, from your findings?

RESEARCH FUNDING

Research funding can be obtained in several ways, although not all nurse researchers require financial assistance as some R.G.N. programmes and virtually all undergraduate degree programmes require students to submit a research proposal or carry out a small research project.

Some Regional Health Authorities fund nursing research posts which experienced qualified nurses may apply for. These posts are often funded so as to provide for the investigation of a specific area which has been identified by the Health Authority, so that the nurse has little freedom to choose the area of her work.

It is sometimes possible for employed nurses to negotiate study leave with pay in order to pursue a research project.

Funding can be obtained by approaching:

1 Nursing Research Units such as those at Surrey University, Edinburgh University, Chelsea College or Manchester University.
2 Associations such as the British Diabetic Association, who will sometimes fund research if it will be of benefit to those suffering from the disease.
3 Firms producing drugs or medical equipment as they need knowledge which may support the sale of their products or suggest a need for new products.
4 DHSS institutions such as the Health Education Council (now Authority).
5 There are Trust funds for research such as The Nuffield Provincial Hospital Trust, The Nuffield Foundation, King Edward's Hospital Fund for London.
6 Statutory bodies sponsor research on occasions, as a preparation for major reports or when implementing change.

Before approaching any authority for funding, it would be necessary to submit a research proposal stating the identified problem, the (null) hypothesis (using the literature search as a basis for justification), and the proposed methodology.

THE ETHICAL DIMENSIONS OF A RESEARCH PROJECT

The general topic of ethics in nursing will be considered more fully in a future chapter. However, at this stage it is relevant to list some questions which any nurse researcher should ask herself before starting any study or experiment which involves people:

1 Are the aims and purpose of this research such that it could be of long-term benefit in health care?
2 Will this research cause any unnecessary risks to patients and/or staff?
3 Can I be sure that I will at all times be able to respect confidentiality and maintain anonymity, if I have undertaken to do so?
4 Am I competent to carry out this piece of research?
5 How do I intend to use these research findings?

All health districts in the UK have an ethics committee and any potential nurse researcher wishing to use patients as the subjects of her study would have to present such a committee with a research proposal outlining the purpose and methodology of her intended work. Without the approval of the relevant committee, nursing research involving the use of patients/clients cannot proceed.

It is the first duty of the researcher that research shall do the participant no harm.

Norton (1975)

To achieve maximum validity, the researcher should draw on primary sources of information such as *On Trained Nursing for the Sick Poor* (Nightingale 1876), The Platt report (1975), the Briggs report (1972), rather than referring to secondary sources such as C. Woodham-Smith's *Florence Nightingale* (1960) or Monica Baly's *Nursing and Social Change* (1980).

READING A RESEARCH REPORT

Having considered the writing of a research report, you may now have developed a heightened awareness of critical questions which you should ask yourself when reading a report.

Remember, not all research studies have been published: there are many unpublished pieces of work lying dormant in university, college and nursing school libraries. An example of this is the Steinberg collection at the Royal College of Nursing.

Remember, also, that the fact of publication does not guarantee that the results of an investigation are either valid or reliable.

SOME INITIAL CRITICAL QUESTIONS

1 What is the study about?
— Is there an abstract or summary?
— Does the title of the report accurately reflect the problem studied?
— Was the study historical, experimental or descriptive in its approach?
— What assessment can be made from the way the study is presented as to its quality and to its relevance to your field of work? E.g. chapter or section headings; appendices; references?

2 Why was the study carried out?
— Was the purpose of the study worthwhile?
— Who asked for it?
— Who paid for it?
— How were the results to be used?

3 Who was the investigator?
— Was he or she qualified to carry out this type of study?
— Was it the first piece of research the investigator had carried out?
— Did he or she have adequate support and resources?

MORE DETAILED QUESTIONS

THE RESEARCH REPORT
A research report consists of three basic parts:

1 A statement of the subject or problem under investigation.
2 An explanation of the methodology, that is the research design and procedures used in carrying out the research.
3 An analysis of the data and a report of the findings on which the conclusions and recommendations are based.

Where appropriate, the following points should be considered:

THE SUBJECT OF THE INVESTIGATION:

1 What was the research problem?
— Is the problem placed within the framework of existing theory or knowledge; is it clearly related to previous research?

2 Why was this problem selected for study?
— Had any relevant research been carried out before?
— Was the literature search adequate?
— Did the literature suggest ideas or tools relevant to the planned study?

THE RESEARCH DESIGN

3 What hypotheses were tested or how were the objectives defined?
— Are the hypotheses/objectives stated clearly?
— Are they derived from previous research?
— Are definitions given and are they clear and concise?
— Are any assumptions stated and are they justified?

4 What kind of information was collected?
— What population was selected for the study – of people? events?
— How was the sample selected?
— Does the method of obtaining the sample seem appropriate?
— Was the sample large enough?
— Was the sample representative of the population and unbiased?
— Were there any variables or factors which were pertinent to the study which were not included?

5 How was the information collected?
— What instruments or tools were used?
— How were they tested? Was there a pilot study?
— Were the instruments used valid – that is, did they measure what they were supposed to measure?
— Were the instruments used reliable – could they be used again with the same kind of results?

6 How were the data analysed?
— Were the results analysed by computer or by 'hand'?
— Were the appropriate statistical tests used?

THE RESULTS

7 What were the main results of the study?
— Were the objectives met?
— Were the hypotheses accepted or rejected?
— Are there discrepancies between information presented in tables and graphs and that in the text of the article?
— Are the data clearly presented?

CONCLUSIONS

8 What are the implications of the study?

—   Is the discussion clearly separate from the actual findings?

—   Are the investigators' interpretations based on the data?

EVALUATION

9 What comments/criticisms should be made about the methods, results and conclusions?

—   Is the work clearly presented?

—   Is the report logical and well organized?

FURTHER STUDY

1   Having identified a possible area for nursing research perhaps you could use this, or any other identified problem, to write a research proposal.

2   Find a piece of research which was published within the last six months.

    Use the above check-list to respond to the critical questions.

3   When you have read Chapter 5, 'Ethical and Legal Issues in Nursing Practice', return to this chapter and decide whether the methodology proposed to evaluate pressure sore treatment would have been ethically justifiable.

REFERENCES

Baly, M. E. 1980. *Nursing and Social Change*. William Heinemann Medical Books Ltd., London.

Briggs, A. 1972. *The Report of the Committee on Nursing*. HMSO, London.

Clark, J. Macleod. 1981. Communication in nursing. *Nursing Times*, 1 January, Vol.77, No.1, pp.12–18.

Henderson, V. 1969. The basic principles of nursing care. International Council of Nurses, Geneva.

Huff, D. 1975. *How to Lie With Statistics*. Penguin, London.

Iles, J. E. M. and Newman, S. 1975. Intravenous therapy problems encountered by nurses. *Nursing Times*. 15 May, Vol.71, pp.767–9.

Nightingale, F. 1876. *On Trained Nursing for the Sick Poor*. (Cited in C. Woodham-Smith below.)

Norton, D. 1957. *Looking after Old People at Home*. Council of Social Service, London.

Norton, D. 1975. *An investigation of geriatric nursing problems*. Churchill Livingstone, Edinburgh.

Platt, H. 1983. The welfare of children in hospital. *Report of the Committee*. DHSS, London.

Rowntree, 1981. *Statistics Without Tears*. Penguin, London.

UKCC, 1986. *Project 2000 – A New Preparation for Practice*. UKCC, London.

Woodham-Smith, C. 1960. *Florence Nightingale*. Constable, London.

ETHICAL AND LEGAL ISSUES IN NURSING PRACTICE

CONTENTS

What is moral philosophy?   83
The personal ethic   85
The professional ethic   85

Identifying ethical dilemmas   87

Strategies for resolving ethical dilemmas   89
Curtin's ethical decision-making model   89
Bergman's ethical decision-making model   91

Legal aspects of nursing practice   92
Liability for accidents   92
Care of property   93
Witnessing wills   93
Patient consent to treatment   93

Further study   94

References   95

The UKCC (1985) suggests that two competencies of a nurse are the abilities to:

— demonstrate knowledge and understanding to meet the requirements of legislation which is relevant to his or her practice.

— recognize and uphold the personal and confidential rights of patients and clients.

Each person within the health care setting has legal and moral rights. Clearly the rights of the care giver and those of the client who receives that care will at times conflict.

The aim of this chapter is to give the student an understanding of the relevance of moral philosophy within nursing and to consider some legal aspects of care which may influence any decision-making process.

WHAT IS MORAL PHILOSOPHY?

The term moral philosophy is often used synonymously with the term ethics, and so it shall be throughout this text.

What does the term 'ethics' mean to you?

With colleagues, or on your own, list the ideas or thoughts triggered off in your mind by the use of the word 'ethical'.

You may have listed words such as 'sense of duty', 'obligation', 'good/bad', 'values', 'morals', or you may have thought of medical concepts such as euthanasia, abortion, informed consent.

An attempt to answer the question 'How, all things considered, ought a human being to behave?'

Mary Warnock

This question, posed by Baroness Warnock in 1978, is by no means a new one.

Aristotle referred to 'monumental ethics' as a 'natural law, written in the hearts of men'. Rousseau described moral sense as a 'noble savage' which, he suggested, was innate and develops between the ages of two and eight years. The nineteenth-century moralist Kant advocated a belief in the 'categorical imperative' – we do things because we must and there is no acceptable alternative. Existentialist thinkers such as Sartre defined ethics in terms of decision making; Heiddeger, for example, suggested that ethical decisions are those which are freely made.

However it is described, there is no doubt that the study of ethics has Cognitive, Affective and Behavioural Components.

cognitive Suggests use of the intellect, knowledge, thinking, reasoning.

affective Indicates thought processes based on innate feelings which are influenced by upbringing, socialization, culture, life's experiences, social pressures.

behavioural The behavioural component is the practical element of ethics. It refers to the actions which result from the ethical premises that determine individual actions.

Not all the decisions which we make are rooted in ethics or morality.

When playing a game of tennis with an equal, the chances are that you will obey the rules and play to win. Ethics only enter into this situation if you are playing with a child and, while still obeying the rules, you sometimes purposely allow him to win in order not to destroy his confidence.

Although there is often a close connection between ethics, abiding by the rules, 'doing right', or acting legally, breaking the law may not mean acting unethically.

Can you think of a situation in which this could occur?

A man driving through red traffic lights to get someone to hospital quickly would certainly be breaking the law but would probably not be deemed to be acting unethically.

Conversely, keeping meticulously to the law may mean acting unethically.

Can you suggest any situations when this could occur?

A nurse going off duty promptly while assisting a surgeon in the middle of an operation would be working strictly in accordance with her contract, but may be jeopardizing a patient's safety.

There is also a close connection between ethics and religion although, again, the two are not interchangeable. All great religions have an ethical component but religion is primarily concerned about the belief in the relationship between the nature of man and the nature of God. The ethical component of religion is that which is related to a prescribed code of behaviour. It is perfectly possible, for example, to accept the 'love thy neighbour' ethic of Christianity without believing the rest of the Christian doctrine.

To return to Baroness Warnock's definition of ethics in which the question is raised, 'How ought a human being to behave?' This pre-empts the further question, 'Behaviour to whom, or to what?'

THE PERSONAL ETHIC

Waddington (1977) describes what he calls the Personal Ethic and the Professional Ethic. He suggests that the personal ethic is that component of a human being which develops self-awareness and distinguishes man from other animals.

Can you think of any other elements which may distinguish man from other animals?

This is a fairly difficult exercise, for animals have, as man does, power to communicate 'societal rules', and they have an awareness of changing time and seasons. In contrast you may have suggested that animals lack a conscience, the ability to reason hypothetically, or a highly developed sense of right and wrong. If you have considered these elements then, in fact, you are approaching the idea that it is the ability to think or reason ethically which makes man unique among animals.

Waddington further describes people without a highly developed sense of moral reasoning as being disorganized, unhappy, 'driven in different directions by every wind that blows', and suggests they will never, in Maslow's (1970) terms, achieve the pinnacle of self-actualization.

THE PROFESSIONAL ETHIC

As its name suggests, the professional ethic relates to the ideologies of a whole profession or to the ethics of individuals working within that body. Policies accepted by a whole profession, such as the Codes of Conduct formulated by the Royal College of Nursing and the UKCC are examples of this. The surgeon who has to decide whether or not to allow his assistant to undertake an operation unsupervised is making a professional decision which has ethical implications on a more individual basis.

The professional ethic may also relate to the society or community within which one is employed. An unfortunate example of this is the person who would be prepared to steal from an institution, while regarding it highly unethical to steal from individual people.

Before moving on to define ethical dilemmas and to consider

approaches for the clarification of these, an examination of four different approaches to ethical problems may prove worthwhile. This will increase your awareness of the premise from which you personally argue.

Each of these approaches is concerned with **goals**, **rights** and **duties**.

What do these terms mean to you?

A goal is a state of affairs which is, in itself, desirable. The concept of 'rights' relates to the entitlement of individuals to control their lives. Duties are obligations felt by individuals to act or not to act in given situations.

UTILITARIANISM

The utilitarian approach is that which was extolled by Jeremy Bentham in the eighteenth century. He saw that the goal in any action was to achieve the greatest happiness for as many as possible. The concepts of duties and rights are secondary in this theory.

DUTY-BASED THEORIES

The approach to decision making based on duty is that supported by Kant, who declared that man should 'act only the maxim that you can will to be a universal one'. Some duty-based thinkers centre their decision-making approaches upon the Law of God – the Ten Commandments, for example. The goal in duty-based thinking is of negligible importance as, indeed, are the rights of the individuals involved.

RIGHTS-BASED THEORIES

The goal is equally unimportant for rights-based theorists, such as Thomas Paine who, in the eighteenth century, wrote about the 'Rights of Man'. The United Nations Organization Children's Charter which lists twelve children's rights illustrates this approach to decision making.

INTUITIONALISTS

These consider the goal, the rights and the duties involved in decision making to be of equal importance, and judge the value of each according to the individual situation.

Which type of approach do you think that you adopt when making a decision?

There are, of course, pros and cons for each approach. Can you identify them?

The utilitarian approach may appear very attractive. However, happiness for many may result in unhappiness for the minority and could lead to unethical behaviour. Duty-based theorists have a secure foundation for their decision. This approach can be somewhat inflexible, although it does tend to favour the law abiding. Decisions made in the light of rights-based theories are usually made out of respect for the individuals involved. There must inevitably be some conflict of rights, however, in nearly all situations. Intuitionalists accept the good in each system and tend to take a flexible approach to decision making, leaving room for progress. As with right-based theories, problems arise with conflict between individual intuition and judgement.

Having considered – albeit extremely briefly – four different approaches to the decision-making process, let us now return to my original question, 'what does the term "ethics" mean to you?' What, for instance, makes my decision to play a game of adult tennis non-ethical while the decision to play to allow a child to win is an ethical one?

Indeed, what approach would I be using in making this decision?

Playing to allow a child to win (which, I would suggest, is an intuitionalist approach) involves elements of

| 'doing good' | 'self-sacrifice' |
| 'right' (or wrong!) | 'choosing between people' |

Melia (1987) suggests that allocation of clean sheets when supplies are limited presents an ethical dilemma.

IDENTIFYING ETHICAL DILEMMAS

What is an ethical dilemma? Leah Curtin (1983) clearly identifies the components of an ethical dilemma thus:

(a) it does not solely belong within science;
(b) it is inherently perplexing;
(c) it has implications which touch on many areas of human concern.

Using these criteria, you can perhaps understand my earlier contention that anyone working in the health care setting must surely meet ethical dilemmas every day. I have already referred to Melia's suggestion that the allocation of clean sheets poses an ethical dilemma.

Can you now, using Curtin's criteria, identify why this is so?

Can you also note for yourself any situations in which you feel you have made, or are having to make, ethical decisions?

Let us now consider an everyday occurrence in the life of a student nurse. You are planning your morning's work and have been allocated the following four patients:

Mrs Windsor: An elderly lady who needs feeding. Her breakfast is on her locker, and her cup of tea is getting cold.
Mrs Brown: Who is to have some X-rays taken at 11.30 a.m. She *seems* perfectly fit otherwise.
Mrs French: Who has an intravenous infusion running, which has stopped. She is due to go to the operating threatre in one hour's time.
Mrs Martin: A frail, emaciated elderly lady who has been incontinent of urine and is lying in a wet bed.

What do you do?
Whom do you care for first?
How do you manage?
This may be something you would like to discuss with your colleagues.

Possibly the first conclusions you have reached is that you haven't been given enough information to make any decision, and I would agree with this. You need to assess your own experience and capabilities, and you need to know which staff are working with you. Before making any decision, then, you need to be in full possession of all the relevant facts.

The problem presented here is, surely, an ethical one as it is inherently perplexing, and it does have implications which touch many areas of human concern.

It is possible to argue the case for attending to any of these four ladies first.
Indeed you may like to attempt this exercise.

Mrs Windsor obviously needs her breakfast, and may well not drink her tea if it is cold. Taking into account the importance of adequate nutrition for the elderly, it would be easy to justify the feeding of Mrs Windsor first.

It would be equally valid to argue the case for seeing Mrs Brown first. She may seem 'perfectly fit', but unless someone makes time to talk and listen to her, many very real worries and fears could remain unresolved.

Mrs French's intravenous infusion has stopped running. This could, in some circumstances, present you with a life-threatening situation – one which you may feel you should deal with immediately.

Your knowledge about effects of urine on skin, particularly that of a frail, emaciated, elderly lady, may make you think that you should initially care for Mrs Martin.

I cannot offer you a 'right' or 'wrong' answer, because there is none, and this is possibly why establishing priorities for care can prove to be such a difficult task. Patient allocation, individual patient care and the planning of that care present nurses with ethical dilemmas wherever they are working. We are again talking about the allocation of resources, and the fact that, whilst you are caring for one person, you are denying another your attention.

It is, perhaps, interesting that, whilst the problem I presented you with does not solely belong within science, certainly an element of scientific knowledge (i.e. the nutritional needs of an elderly person, the action of urine on the skin) is necessary for the clarification of the dilemma.

STRATEGIES FOR RESOLVING ETHICAL DILEMMAS

Having worked through this problem once, perhaps you could do so again using an ethical decision-making model, see below.

CURTIN'S ETHICAL DECISION-MAKING MODEL (see fig. 5.1)

Stage one. Is this an ethical dilemma? The elements which certain considered inherent in an ethical dilemma have been listed on page 87. Having identified these elements, you could clarify the situation further by answering the following questions:
(a)   Is this a case of conflicting rights?
(b)   Are duties conflicting with the outcomes?
(c)   Is the problem one of lying or withholding the truth?
(d)   Is it a case of powerlessness versus authority?
N.B. **The clearer the definitions, the more precise the analysis.**

Stage two of this model involves the collection of **background information or data base**. The questions you should ask yourself are:
(a)   Who is involved in the situation?
(b)   What information is available (scientific, cultural, sociological, psychological)?
(c)   Information should be gathered, organized and ranked according to its **direct relevance for the decision at hand!**

Stage three. At this point, you need to consider the **individuals involved in decision making**. All persons involved in a particular decision must be identified, together with how they are involved.
(a)   What is the scope of their authority and responsibility?
(b)   On what foundation are their duties asserted?
(c)   How free is a person to make a decision?
(d)   Who should be making the decision and why?

Fig. 5.1 Curtin's ethical decision-making model (Curtin and Flaherty, 1983).

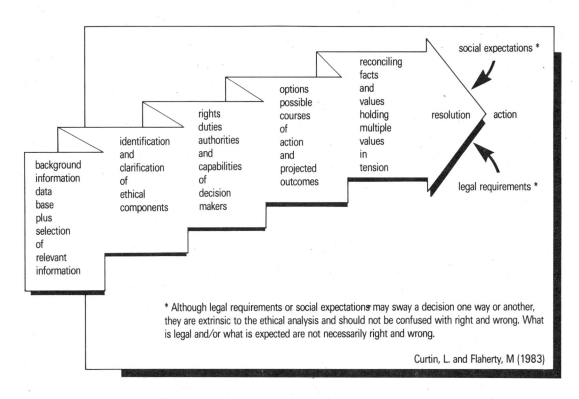

background information data base plus selection of relevant information

identification and clarification of ethical components

rights duties authorities and capabilities of decision makers

options possible courses of action and projected outcomes

reconciling facts and values holding multiple values in tension

social expectations *

resolution — action

legal requirements *

* Although legal requirements or social expectations may sway a decision one way or another, they are extrinsic to the ethical analysis and should not be confused with right and wrong. What is legal and/or what is expected are not necessarily right and wrong.

Curtin, L. and Flaherty, M (1983)

Stage four. Options or possible courses of action. One must project as accurately as possible the consequences of each course of action, and identify the good and/or the harm that can result.

Stage five. Reconciling facts and principles. One must hold various viewpoints, beliefs, values in a creative tension whilst one decides the ranking of the rights and duties involved in the situation. **The reason for the ranking and ultimately the decision itself must be articulated rationally and defended.**

Stage six. Shared decisions and resolution.
(*a*)   Is the problem better solved by one's participation or by one's withdrawal?
(*b*)   Is the situation best handled by submission to the authority of the group?
(*c*)   Should one stand alone as a dissenter?
There will be times, even when a unanimous decision is made, when legal requirements or social expectations or both will sway the final decision.

But remember, neither the law nor social custom is necessarily right and should not be confused with an absolute standard of rightness.

If you have difficulty using this model, return to my discussion of the problem of which of the four patients you should see to first (page 88), and see if you can fit the points which I have raised into any of the six stages of the model as described.

Having completed this exercise, perhaps you could now address yourself to the application of another model of decision making, that designed by the Israeli nurse, Rebecca Bergman, in 1973. The stages of the process of ethical decision making as described by Bergman are listed below.

BERGMAN'S (1973) ETHICAL DECISION-MAKING MODEL (see Fig. 5.2)

There are several steps between encountering an ethical conflict and resolving it:

1 The nurse is faced with the problem. She must identify its major aspects and determine what information is available and what further is required.
2 She then gathers the facts needed to obtain a clear picture of the issues.
3 With more complete knowledge she then reconstructs the situation.
4 This situation is now examined very carefully in the light of her philosophy of life and nursing, as well as her store of scientific knowledge.
5 She studies alternatives for action, and takes a decision.
6 She implements her decisions to the best of her ability.

Fig. 5.2 Flow-chart showing the process of dealing with complex ethical issues (Bergman 1973).

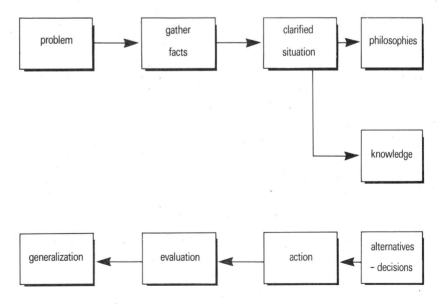

7   She evaluates her decisions and implementation in the light of the results.

8   She adds these findings to her store of general knowledge to be used in similar or related experiences.

You will probably note similarities between the two models, the main differences being that Curtin explicitly recognizes that legal requirements and social expectations will influence any resolution, while Bergman recognizes that at the end of any decision-making process lessons will have been learned and generalizations can be made which will bring experience and knowledge into future situations.

LEGAL ASPECTS OF NURSING PRACTICE

As Curtin's decision-making model explicitly indicates, you must, when making any decision within nursing, consider legal aspects of the situation.

Before continuing any further, you should acquaint yourself with the UKCC Code of Conduct (1986).

In the Civil law this Code is not a legal document, but violation of the Code could lead to a nurse being struck off the Professional Register. The Code embraces the safety, well-being and respect of patients' rights. It also addresses the need to maintain professional competence. Interestingly, it decries the use of professional status in the endorsing of commercial products. When we read, therefore, that 'nurse Jones recommends Brown's Bunion pads' we can afford to be somewhat sceptical!

There are aspects of promoting patient safety, well-being and respect for the individual where the nurse could be legally liable. In this text, we consider a few. These are:

(a)   liability for accidents;
(b)   care of property;
(c)   the witnessing of wills;
(d)   patient consent to treatment.

Of course, there are many other areas where any nurse, either in the community or in hospital, may be legally accountable. The golden rule is probably to 'think before you act', and acquaint yourself with any potential problems which may apply specifically to the area in which you are working.

LIABILITY FOR ACCIDENTS

The key question here is, 'when is a health carer held to be liable following an accident or injury to a patient?'. The general answer is that the complainant has to prove neglect. For example, if all possible precautions are taken to prevent an elderly person from falling and she still falls, then staff are not held to be responsible.

Ward or departmental managers can be called legally to account if they depute junior members of staff to carry out a task for which they are not competent, and they make an error as a result.

To what extent do you think a student nurse should consider herself accountable if she is asked to carry out a task which she feels incompetent to do?

CARE OF PROPERTY

It is important to remember that all national hospitals have been instructed by the Department of Health and Social Security to disclaim responsibility for a patient's belongings, except those that have been handed over to the hospital for safe keeping.

Be certain that you are aware of the policy within your district for the safe storage of property!

Property which had been handed over for safe keeping and subsequently becomes lost is the responsibility of the health authority and the patient can sue.

If a patient dies, then small amounts of money or goods of minor value can generally be handed direct to relatives, who sign a receipt. Larger amounts should, strictly speaking, be handed to executors of a person's will.

Again, check the policy in your district.

WITNESSING WILLS

People in hospital often feel the necessity to make a will. A patient may wish to call his own solicitor to facilitate this, or the hospital may employ one.

If a patient asks you as a nurse to act as a witness to his signature, then as a citizen she is entitled to do so. However, some health authority rules forbid this, so

Check the rules in your area.

PATIENT CONSENT TO TREATMENT

It is a rule of law that no one may wilfully interfere with the body of another person without the consent of that person.

The patient's consent to medical examination, other than internal examination under anaesthetic; to medical treatment, including injections, and to minor surgery such as wound suturing, is ordinarily inferred from his coming to hospital for treatment.

The patient's consent in writing must be obtained before internal examination or any exploratory procedure under anaesthetic takes place.

Any child under sixteen years of age must have a consent form signed by a parent or guardian.

If, in an emergency situation, it is necessary for a doctor to carry out a procedure without obtaining consent (e.g. if the patient is unconscious), then this is permissible to save life.

FURTHER STUDY

1 Identify the ethical components and analyse the following situations using a decision-making model.

SITUATION 1

Mr Williams has carcinoma of the bronchus. His prognosis is very poor. Doctors discuss this with Mr Williams' wife and his daughters. All of these ladies are adamant that Mr Williams should not be told the truth, which is that he only has about six months to live. One day, Mr Williams says to the student nurse who is caring for him, 'I've got cancer, I know it. I'm going to die, aren't I?'.

SITUATION 2

The policy in your district is that nurses do not accept gifts from patients. One day, a patient, who you know has very little income, offers you £2 with the words 'I really want you to have this, to thank you for all you've done for me'.

SITUATION 3

Mrs Anderson is a young lady who is admitted with acute appendicitis. She is very ill, and doctors fear that if they don't operate appendicitis will set in. However, Mrs Anderson is terrified; she will not listen to discussion about the need for surgery. Her husband is a travelling salesman and moves to contact him have been unsuccessful. The registrar suggests administration of a sedative to calm Mrs Anderson, so that he can reason with her about the need to perform this potentially life-saving operation.

2 You should be aware of the legal status of nursing records and care plans (see chapter 2). Why is it so important to avoid use of abbreviations in nursing records?

3 Acquaint yourself with disciplinary procedure. (References to Pyne will help here.)

4 Read the Health and Safety at Work Act (1974). Where do your personal responsibilities lie in relation to this?

REFERENCES

NURSING ETHICS

Beauchamp, T. L. and Childress, J. F. 1983. *Principles of Bio-medical Ethics.* 2nd edition. Oxford University Press, London.

Bergman, R. 1973. Ethics, concepts and practice. *International Nursing Review*, Vol.20, No.5, pp.140, 141, 152.

Curtin, L. and Flaherty, M. 1983. *Nursing Ethics: Theories and Pragmatics.* Robert J. Brady, Bowie, Maryland.

Maslow, A. H. 1970. *Motivation and Personality.* Harper & Row, New York.

Melia, K. 1987. Everyday ethics. *Nursing Times/Nursing Mirror,* Vol.83, No.3, 21 January, pp.28–9.

Thompson, I. E., Melia, K. M. and Boyd, K. 1983. *Nursing Ethics.* Churchill Livingstone, Edinburgh.

Waddington, C. H. 1977. *Tools for Thought.* Paladin, William Collins, London.

Warnock, M. 1978. *Ethics since 1900.* Oxford University Press, London.

LEGAL ASPECTS OF NURSING

Alleway, Lyn. 1986. Conduct unbecoming. *Nursing Times & Mirror.* 12 March, pp.19–20.

Carson, D. 1987. Negligence – defining responsibility. *Professional Nurse* 2 (5), February, pp.141–5.

Dimond, B. 1987a. Doing the right thing. *Nursing Times & Mirror.* 85, 4 February, p.61.

Dimond, B. 1987b. Your disobedient servant: legal implications of the nurse/client. *Nursing Times & Mirror.* 82, 21 January, pp.28–31.

H.M.S.O. 1974. *The Health and Safety at Work Act.* HMSO, London.

Mawson, D. 1986. Seeking informed consent. *Nursing Times & Mirror.* 82, 5 February, pp.52–3.

Murchison, I. 1982. *Nursing and the Law: Legal Accountability in the Nursing Process.* C. V. Mosby, Missouri.

Pyne, R. 1985. Disciplinary process. *Senior Nurse* (2), 23 January, pp.7–10.

Pyne, R. 1987. What's your verdict? *Senior Nurse* 6(3), March, pp.15–16.

U.K.C.C. 1986. *Project 2000 – A New Preparation for Practice.*

Vousden, M. 1987. When a nightmare becomes a reality. *Nursing Times & Mirror*, February, pp.28–30.

Young, A. P. 1981. *Legal Problems in Nursing Practice.* Harper & Row, New York.

PART TWO

EDITH AND ALBERT BAKER

Albert has Alzheimer's disease and is admitted to hospital following an accident at home.

Caring for an ill person at home for a long while will require great resources of care, compassion and good health on the part of the 'carer'. Such care giving can be both emotionally and physically exhausting. The majority of the carers are women, and their task is formidable.

Bring to mind the elderly confused patients you have nursed in elderly care and general wards, or in the community. What did you learn from the experience?

CHECK ▶

Make sure you understand and investigate the following before completing the study questions in this vignette:

1 ▶ The effects on behaviour and personality of Alzheimer's disease (dementia of the elderly). (See page 102 for key references on this condition).

2 ▶ The surgical treatment and nursing care needed by an elderly person with a fractured femur.

Edith and Albert Baker have been married for forty years. They met each other in 1946 just after the war ended. They both worked in local government throughout their working lives and used their spare time gardening and going on caravanning holidays in England and France. The Bakers did not have children. In this way they shared work and leisure time interests throughout their lives.

Their circumstances changed five years ago when Mr Baker's behaviour and personality began to change. He became unable to remember recent events and became angry over seemingly minor events and frustrations. He would refuse to go to work, and would leave early, and the quality of his work rapidly deteriorated. It was then that Mr Baker was diagnosed as having Alzheimer's disease and retired from work. Mrs Baker took the opportunity to retire early too, after being counselled by her GP about the nature and the probable development of Mr Baker's illness.

Recently, caring for Mr Baker has become a full-time occupation. Mrs Baker accepts this as being her responsibility, and has been coping unsupported. Mr Baker needs to be told what to do throughout the day, otherwise his wife has found that he stays in bed or sits in an armchair or paces up and down all day without dressing or washing himself, or seeing the need to eat.

On the day Mr Baker fell and fractured his femur, Mrs Baker had spent about ten minutes out of the house. She had gone to the post box and had been stopped by her neighbour for a chat. He was found lying in the hall at the foot of the stairs when she walked in the front door.

Elderly people experience falls for a number of reasons, and the effects of such falls can be far reaching. For a discussion of this topic see Smith, C. (1985) and Batehup and Squires (1986).

In the Accident and Emergency department of the District General Hospital Mr Baker was examined and X-rays were taken of his legs and skull. He was calm, he did not speak, but he allowed these examinations to take place. He had fractured the shaft of his left femur and this needed to be treated by internal fixation using a pin and plate. Overnight, skin traction was to be applied, and the following afternoon Mr Baker was to be prepared for surgery.

If you were a nurse in the orthopaedic ward Mr Baker was transferred to that evening, and all the information you had was that the patient was 66 years old, male, with a fractured left femur and Alzheimer's disease, how would you set about admitting and assessing him when he arrived? (See Briscoe 1983 and Versluysen 1986.)

Your assessment would have been made with the assistance of Mrs Baker and you would have taken particular note of Mr Baker's needs in relation to the activities of living such as eating and drinking, sleeping and communication. You would have planned the care he needed to ensure that the fracture was immobilized and that he was free of pain.

Mrs Baker left the ward at 9 p.m. She had spent much of her time that evening telling her husband where he was and what had happened to him. Mr Baker was able to use a urinal and drank some tea and hot chocolate, although he would not eat. When Mrs Baker had gone, he became restless and started shouting 'Oi, oi, oi' and banging the bedtable against his locker.

If you were the nurse coming on night duty at this point when Baker is noisy and restless, what would you assess about the situation Mr Baker is in, and what strategies would you plan to try out? (See Brooking 1986).

The goals for Mr Baker's post-operative care are that he should recover from the surgery and the anaesthetic safely and without post-operative complications developing. Since it becomes clear that he is unable to co-operate with deep breathing and leg exercises to minimize the probability of developing a chest infection or deep-veined thrombosis, he receives extra physiotherapy instead, and it is planned to mobilize him on the first day after surgery if he is well enough. Mr Baker accepts the care given him by the physiotherapist and he does not seem concerned about his intravenous infusion or his wound drain.

Mrs Baker arrives on the ward during the afternoon of the first post-operative day. She asks the Ward Sister about her husband's progress, and the Sister expresses concern that the ward staff are unable to get Mr Baker to eat and she asks for Mrs Baker's advice.

It is at this point, in recounting her own methods of trying to ensure that her husband eats, that Mrs Baker starts weeping.

How would you behave if you were with Mrs Baker at this point? (See Tschudin 1982. Also Taylor 1987 for a personal account of caring for someone with Alzheimer's disease).

The ward sister encourages Mrs Baker to express her worries about her husband, not just about helping him eat but in the wider context of coping generally. It is clear that she is finding his need of constant care an ever-increasing burden. The Sister gives her plenty of time to express these difficult feelings.

Two nurses help Mr Baker get out of bed the following day, and he walks round his bed before sitting in a chair. Mrs Baker brings in some home-made Cornish pasties, one of which is heated in the ward kitchen. Mr Baker eats this and asks for another. Mrs Baker sits with him and they both have a cup of tea.

Jane Reynolds, the ward's social worker, comes to see them to discuss the care and support that can be offered to them both. (For methods of helping carers of dependent relatives, see MacGuire and Pearson 1987, Tyler 1987 and Garrett 1985).

DISCUSSION AND FURTHER STUDY

Mr Baker was transferred later in the week to an elderly care ward which ensured that his rehabilitation and recovery from his fractured femur were focused on, and his dementia was catered for by competent staff in an environment which was primed to maintain and enhance the dignity of patients and minimize the effects of hospitalization. Mrs Baker was put in touch with the Alzheimer's Disease Society which had a group in her locality. The elderly care ward team operated a system of 'respite care' beds, and plans were made to support Mrs Baker whilst she continued to care for her husband.

1   One of the ways in which elderly people who are confused and disorientated can be helped is by 'reality orientation' (see Clarke 1987).

2   Some nursing research has assessed the effects of different lighting levels on the behaviour of confused and disorientated patients (Fox , Ford, Fitch and Donovan 1987).

3   Resources available for the support and assistance of those caring for relatives and friends who need constant surveillance and nursing care are outlined in the literature produced by the Health Education Authority, for example the booklet CA 80, *'Who Cares?'*

Investigate the local resources available in your Health District for those caring for heavily dependent people.

---

4   Elderly people may be seen as unpopular and unco-operative; this may be the result of difficulties encountered by nurses in communicating skilfully with them. Being able to communicate with elderly people who are confused and disorientated is challenging and needs creativity and skill. (See Fielding 1981 and Macleod Clark 1986).

REFERENCES TO VIGNETTE 1

KEY REFERENCES

Brooking, J. I. 1986. Dementia and confusion in the elderly. In Redfern, S. J. (ed.) *Nursing Elderly People*. Churchill Livingstone, Edinburgh.

Ferry, G. 1987. The genetic roots of dementia. *New Scientist*, 113, 12 March, pp.20–1.

Hudson, B. 1984. Who cares for the carers? *Health and Social Service Journal*, 5 July, pp.790–1.

Smith, P. and Leigh, N. 1986. The biology of ageing: the ageing brain. *Geriatric Nursing and Home Care*. November/December, pp.20–1, 23–5.

ADDITIONAL REFERENCES

Batehup, L. and Squires, A. 1986. Mobility. In Redfern, S. J. (ed.) *Nursing Elderly People*. Churchill Livingstone, Edinburgh.

Briscoe, S. 1983. Nursing care study. Fractured femur. *Nursing Mirror*. 29 June, pp.50–53.

Clark, J. Macleod 1986. Communication with elderly people. In Redfern, S. J. (ed.) *Nursing Elderly People*. Churchill Livingstone, Edinburgh.

Clarke, C. 1987. Reaching for reality. *Nursing Times*, 29 July, pp.24–7.

Fielding, P. 1981. Communicating with geriatric patients. In Bridge, W. and Macleod Clark, J. (eds.) *Communication in Nursing Care*. HM & M Publishers Ltd, London.

Fox, J., Ford, M., Fitch, S. and Donovan, A. 1987. Light in the darkness. *Nursing Times*. 7 January, pp.26–9.

Garrett, G. 1985. Pensions and benefits for the elderly and their carers. *Professional Nurse*, I(2), November, pp.45–6.

MacGuire, J. and Pearson, J. 1987. A welcome break. *Nursing Times*. 12 August, pp.48–50.

Smith, C. 1985. Trauma in the elderly. *Nursing Mirror*. 17 July, pp.36–9.

Taylor, P. 1987. A living bereavement. *Nursing Times*. 29 July, pp.27–30.

Tschudin, V. 1982. *Counselling Skills for Nurses*. Baillière Tindall, London.

Tyler, J. 1987. Give us a break. *Nursing Times*. 16 December, pp.32–5.

Versluysen, M. 1986. How elderly patients with femoral fracture develop pressure sores in hospital. *British Medical Journal*, 292, 17 May, pp.1311–13.

LISA BARRATT

Lisa has Down's syndrome and is cared for by her family.

The birth of a child is a time of great excitement. It's also a time of upheaval. Once there is a new member of the family, life can never be exactly the same again. If the child is born with any form of disability, the readjustment which the family have to make is that much greater.

Do you know of any child who has a physical or mental disability? To what extent is family life enhanced or complicated by this child?

CHECK ▶

Make sure you understand and investigate the following before completing the study questions in this vignette:

1 ▶ What is meant by the term Down's syndrome?

2 ▶ Stages of a 'normal' child's development. See key references on page 109 information on these topics.

Chris and Jane Barratt were delighted when their child was born as they had both longed for a daughter. They already had two sons aged 9 and 5 years. Lisa was born following a normal pregnancy and labour. A few hours after the birth the doctor confirmed that she had Down's syndrome.

By recalling to mind any children you have met with Down's syndrome, or from your reading, can you say how the doctor would have made this diagnosis? Cunningham 1982 will help you here.

Down's syndrome is usually detectable at birth, but occasionally the defect is not noticed for a few days after birth. The signs and features of a child with Down's syndrome are clearly identifiable. The major ones are: distinctive slanting eyes; a single crease across the palms of the hand; a large, often protruding, tongue and sparse, dry, light-coloured hair. Children with Down's syndrome often have abnormalities of the respiratory tract and heart. Many used to die young, although improved surgery today offers a better prognosis.

Chris and Jane are very distressed initially, and really don't understand how this has happened to them, as there is no history of Down's syndrome in the family.

What explanation can you give to them? (See Cunningham 1982.)

They need to know that the chromosomes act as the 'biological blueprint' which carry the genes of the individual. Sometimes these are damaged, broken or muddled in some way so that from conception the biological programme for building the cells for the new human being is faulty. Chromosome abnormalities may be inherited, but they also occur randomly; the risk does increase as the mother ages. 'Normal' children have 23 matching pairs of chromosomes in every cell. A child with Down's syndrome typically has an extra chromosome in the 21st pair making a total of 47, although other abnormal arrangements in the chromosomes have been identified.

Even though they've been given some explanation as to the cause of Down's syndrome, Chris and Jane are obviously still distressed.

What emotions do you think they may experience at this time? (For a consideration of the grieving process, see Kubler-Ross 1980.)

Their feelings might include extreme feelings of shock, helplessness, shame, embarrassment and guilt. They could even feel frustrated and reject the child. This may be seen as part of the process of grief and mourning for the normal child who was never born. They could equally be in a state of chronic sorrow because they're faced with the life-long reality of the situation. The mother of a handicapped child is often denied that glow of pride which others experience. She may resent the pity she receives and is unlikely to wish to be overwhelmed by feelings of sympathy. Most people with normal children experience embarrassment in their encounters with the mother and her handicapped child.

Like many parents, Jane and Christopher want to know as much as possible from the start, yet they need time to discuss the same facts many times before they can grasp their full significance. These should therefore be explained as simply as possible.

Chris and Jane did not reject their daughter. After the initial shock they decided to keep her at home and Jane decided to give up work so that she could look after Lisa herself.

What government agencies are there to give support to parents such as Chris and Jane?

Obviously the largest statutory helping agency is the National Health Service and within this Chris and Jane will be able to make use of the services of the general practitioner, the health visitor, speech therapists, physiotherapists, occupational therapists, and possibly clinical psychologists.

1 SOCIAL SERVICES DEPARTMENT

Social Services Departments were first set up in 1948 on a local basis. Their concern is with various people who for one reason or another have a wide range of problems which may include poverty, poor housing, sickness, injury, old age and physical and mental handicaps. In other words, all those people who have need of help and support from the general community. Social Services Departments administrate government legislation which relates to those people with special problems.

2 EDUCATION SERVICES

Since 1970, the responsibility for the education of children with any form of disability has rested with the Education Department instead of the Health Authority.

3 SELF-HELP GROUPS

In addition to government support, there are self-help groups, specifically the Down's Children's Association and ADB (Aid for Down's Babies), based in Edinburgh.

Jane is closely supported in caring for Lisa by the health visitor.

What role do you think the health visitor has in working with the mother and daughter?

When working with parents it is easy to adopt an advisory role which may make parents feel their opinions are being discounted and their experience with the child belittled. Parents are the primary agents of care, and it is they who ultimately have to shoulder the weight of responsibility for the child. Theirs is a long-term commitment, and their own lives will be affected by any decisions made. Chris and Jane have already had to make many adjustments to their lives; thus their views concerning any decisions must always be respected. It is probably true to say that they are the only true experts about their child and their circumstances. So their perceptions of the family's problems are crucial in any discussions that are held about the child.

The health visitor's role, then, may be seen to be one of an objective viewer. Jane is, for example, at times over protective towards Lisa, perhaps due to a misplaced sense of care where she is trying to overcompensate for all the child lacks in life. Her health visitor realizes that this care-taking role sometimes completely dominates Jane's life. This is possibly as a result of Jane's guilt that she is somehow the cause of her child's problems. The health visitor is slightly concerned that Lisa may be unable to attain the independence and mastery of skills which could otherwise be possible.

The health visitor also has an important role in sharing her expertise. She is aware of resources which are available to Jane, Christopher and Lisa.

Perhaps you could consider what resources are available for couples like Jane and Chris.

Your local DHSS Department will have leaflets concerning financial assistance. Your local Social Services Department should have a directory of services available. The Patients Association produces a directory of National Organizations concerned with various diseases and handicaps which is called Self-Help and the Patient. It is published by Gee & Son Limited. Another very useful resource would be your local Citizens Advice Bureau.

It should not be assumed that all children with Down's syndrome have severe learning difficulties. In conjunction with the health visitor Jane does manage to develop Lisa's independence and she takes her first steps at the age of eighteen months. By the age of two she is saying her first words.

Using your knowledge of child development, how near 'the norm' is Lisa at this stage? (See Sheridan 1975.)

The Barratt family is fortunate in that there is a playgroup attached to the local children's Assessment Centre and at two and a half Lisa is able to attend this and play with children with similar problems. At three and a half she is able to attend the local day school for children with severe learning difficulties. She is placed on the intensive remedial language programme so that by the age of seven Lisa has attained a reading age of six years. She can count up to twenty and add up numbers to ten by using counters.

Despite these very positive initiatives, life is not plain sailing for the Barratt family.

What problems as a family unit do you think the Barratts may encounter? (See Abbott 1982.)

Having a child with a disability within the family can affect relationships between parents and other brothers and sisters. At times Chris and Jane feel that the worry and anxiety caused by making decisions about Lisa infringes upon the joy of their marriage; might indeed even lead to complete breakdown. When Chris comes home from work, on occasions Jane seems to have little emotional responsiveness left.

Conversely, there are times when they feel that caring for Lisa has further united the family. They have always shared decision making and the brothers are equally involved in any discussion about Lisa's progress. This means that the Barratts have become a reliant and self-supportive unit.

However, at times Jane's brothers experience feelings of shame and embarrassment at the looks and behaviour of Lisa. They feel, too, that they are expected to be more responsible than friends of the same age. It often seems to them that Jane spends all her time caring for Lisa and has no time for them.

A sensitive health visitor could monitor this and point problems out tactfully to Jane when it seems necessary.

The Warnock Committee was set up by the Ministry of Education in 1974 to review the educational provision for all handicapped children. This committee's essential task was seen as one of considering how teaching and learning could be brought about with children who have a variety of obstacles which impede their progress. Its findings supported the trend towards integrating handicapped with non-handicapped pupils in ordinary schools where possible. Indeed, ten years later government thinking reinforces this concept.

Identify the elements of this concept which could precipitate an ethical dilemma. This may be something you would like to discuss with your colleagues.

The outlook for Lisa, in fact, is bright. There is a slow-learner unit for children with moderate learning difficulties attached to a nearby ordinary school. It is Jane's and Chris's intention to send Lisa there. With help and support from the right teacher, she may make steady, albeit slow, educational progress. Hopefully, too, she will become more socially confident. It is aimed and projected that by the age of eleven Lisa should have a reading age of eight and she should be eligible for the slow-learner unit attached to the local comprehensive school.

The future worries Chris and Jane. Lisa will probably be able to cope with a limited range of social activities but her peers will outstrip her socially and educationally and they will have vocational aims which she will not be able to realize. As an adult, she may be able to find work in a sheltered workshop, or perhaps attend an adult training centre. This may work well as long as she can live at home, but if Jane and Chris should die before Lisa does, then who will care for her?

Many children with Down's syndrome reach a learning plateau at about twelve years. So that, despite Lisa's early encouraging progress, she will probably stick at a certain point. Her movements remain unco-ordinated due to flaccid muscle tone (hypotonia), and her typically over-large tongue means that she will always have speech difficulties. On a positive note, despite intermittent frustrations Lisa is generally a contented young lady.

DISCUSSION AND FURTHER STUDY

In this vignette we have looked at the problems of a family in which one member has a disability.

We have explored the fact that such a disability has effects that are far reaching and require positive confrontation and handling.

In completing this vignette you may like to go on to study further:

1 Other government reports relating to education and facilities available for the mentally and physically disabled in the community.
2 Look at the specific needs available in your local health authority and near your home. What education facilities are there available for children like Lisa?
3 Attempt to analyse the following situation and pin-point the ethical components: Jane is amazed to find that she is expecting their fourth child. In view of her history, an aminocentesis test is performed, as Down's syndrome is a congenital disorder which can be detected in utero. The test is positive and, 16 weeks pregnant, Jane is faced with the dilemma of whether to have the pregnancy terminated or not.

REFERENCES TO VIGNETTE 2

KEY REFERENCES

Abbott, T. 1982. Diverse Report: Problems faced by parents caring for mentally handicapped children at home. *Nursing Times & Mirror*, 5 March, pp.47–9.

Carr, J. 1980. *Helping Your Handicapped Child: A Step by Step Guide to Everyday Problems*. Penguin, London.

Cunningham, C. 1982. *Down's Syndrome: An Introduction for Parents*. Souvenir Press (Condor), London.

Newson, E. and Hipgrave, T. 1982. *Getting Through to Your Handicapped Child*. Cambridge University Press, London.

Sheridan, M. 1975. *From Birth to Five Years: Children's Developmental Progress*. N.F.E.R., Nelson, London.

Warnock, M. 1978. *Special Education Needs. Report of the Committee of Enquiry into the Education of Handicapped Children and Young People*. (Warnock Report). D.E.S.S., London.

ADDITIONAL REFERENCES

Kubler-Ross, E. 1980. Dealing with Death and Dying. In Chaney, P.S. (ed.) *A Nursing Skillbook*. International Communications Inc., Welsh Rd., Horsham.

ERIC BROWN

Eric is having treatment for cancer of the lung.

Cancer is a common cause of ill health, and at present the second most common cause of death in England and Wales. Within the body cancer affects most organs, and each type of cancer has its own natural history. The ability to detect and diagnose different types of cancer varies, as does the means by which they are controlled or cured. We focus here on one type of cancer, cancer of the lung, and one form of treatment, radiotherapy.

What have been your experiences of cancer? How do you think these experiences affect the way in which you approach this topic for study, and indeed the way in which you approach patients who have cancer?

CHECK ▶

Make sure you understand and investigate the following before completing the study question in this vignette, using the key references on page 114 to help you:

1 ▶ The meanings of:
   (a)   carcinogenesis
   (b)   metastases
   (c)   bronchoscopy

2 ▶ Lung cancer, its causes, incidence, treatment and prevention.

Eric Brown is 63 years old and has been a foreman with London Transport Vehicle Maintenance Division for the past forty years. He has never experienced bouts of illness and considers himself to be a fairly fit person, that is until he noticed, last autumn, that he was coughing up more phlegm than usual first thing in the morning, and that he became breathless if he needed to hurry to the tube station. He put these problems down to advancing years and also, reluctantly, to his cigarette smoking. He was a forty-a-day man and had been since the Second World War.

In January he caught a cold which persisted for a couple of weeks.

He found he could not rest at night because of his cough and he found himself to be rather breathless and wheezy even when not exerting himself. Consequently he called into his general practitioner's surgery on his way home from work and was given a prescription for some antibiotics to 'sort out' the chest infection diagnosed by his doctor.

However, since he still felt unwell and dyspnoeic after a week, he returned to see his doctor. This time the doctor made an appointment for him to have a chest X-ray at the local hospital and a consultation with a chest physician. The chest X-ray revealed an abnormal opacity in his lungs, and he was asked to return to the hospital the following week to be admitted for a bronchoscopy.

Mr Brown told the nurse assessing him on admission that he had a 'shadow on his lung' and that he had come in for a special test to find out what it was.

Mr Brown also says he is worried about what is to happen to him. How would you help him overcome his anxiety? (See Wilson-Barnett 1979, especially the chapters on 'The experience of a special test' and 'Reactions to malignant disease and to death and bereavement'.)

Mr Brown undergoes bronchoscopy and a biopsy taken then reveals that he has squamous cell carcinoma of the bronchus (cancer of the lung).

The following day his doctor spends time with him, listening to him and explaining his diagnosis and possible forms of treatment. Although at the beginning of the conversation the doctor uses the word 'shadow' just as Mr Brown does, later on, in response to Mr Brown asking if the 'shadow' is in fact cancer, the doctor replies that it is.

This brief outline of the doctor explaining, truthfully, the diagnosis to Mr Brown, may not reflect your own experiences of the way information about the diagnosis of cancer is shared by health care professionals and patients. You may like to investigate this issue of communication with cancer patients. A description of a research study and a review of some of the literature about communication with cancer patients is given in Bond 1983.

Reading Bond's work, following up some of her references, and others you come across in studying this subject, may help you understand the complexity of the process of communication in situations where patients have 'difficult' diagnoses.

Mr Brown's tumour is not considered to be treatable with surgery (see Mumford 1983). Instead he is to be given a course of radiotherapy treatment over a period of four weeks (see Taylor 1983). His treatment is to start whilst he is an in-patient.

Mr Brown's son Brian arrives just as the doctor is drawing the discussion to a close. The doctor leaves and Mr Brown explains what the 'shadow' is and the treatment that is proposed.

Write down what you would aim to teach Mr Brown about his treatment before he leaves the ward.

Make a note of the activities you would plan and the resources you would use. You may find the following publications useful: Walker 1982, Holmes 1986 and Yasko 1982.

Mr Brown completes his course of treatment. Although he feels tired and becomes depressed towards the end of the four weeks and for the three months following, he copes with this and begins to feel better than he had done in the months prior to his initial hospitalization.

However, some nine months after his treatment finishes his dyspnoea returns. This time it is accompanied by some pain and general discomfort in his chest. Mr Brown's GP refers him to the out-patient department at the hospital earlier than his booked appointment. A chest X-ray shows that he appears to have many small areas of metastases in both lungs and a pleural effusion. Mr Brown is admitted to an acute medical ward straight from out-patients.

Mr Brown's nursing assessment, summarized, is as follows:

◊ Is alert and orientated, and although dyspnoeic is able to talk.

◊ Has explained that he has been admitted so that fluid can be 'taken off' his lung to improve his breathing. He says he is not 'beaten yet'.

◊ Dyspnoeic on exertion. Has been doing activities slowly at home, has not been out of the home for the past week. Is still able to walk up the stairs. His chest pain is constant, like 'toothache'.

◊ He says he is 'skin and bone'. Weight down ten kilos since previous admission. Says he has no appetitie. Mouth moist and clean. Dentures a bit loose fitting now.

◊ No problems with micturition. Bowels now tend to be constipated. Is concerned about this. Last bowel movement three days ago. Normal pattern for the last six months, bowels opened every three or four days.

◊ Hygiene and grooming very good. Manages all needs on his own. No evidence of pressure sore development.

◊ Apyrexial.

◊ Mobile – slowed down due to dyspnoea.

◊ Reads and watches TV. Unable to tend his garden for the past five months. Is planning what is to be done in the garden next year by his son.

◊ Concerned about his increasing dependence on his daughter-in-law who he feels has quite enough 'babies' of her own to look after (son – six months old, two daughters three and seven years.) Says he feels 'pretty useless' now.

◊ Says he sleeps about six or seven hours with three pillows and the window open.

◊ Talked about having cancer, how it suddenly 'caught up' with him. He hopes that once the fluid is removed he will breathe more easily. Said he wanted to get back home.

Write down a plan of care to be discussed with Mr Brown. Nursing strategies for overcoming some of his problems are discussed in Sofaer 1984, *Nursing, 2nd edition of first series* (chronic pain); Brown et al 1986, Foote et al 1986 (breathlessness); Hanks 1983, *Nursing, 20th edition of 3rd series* (advanced cancer); Janes 1986.

In addition to deciding treatment, another important assessment which needs to be made at this point concerns Mr Brown's immediate family support and what plans should be made for his care, as he may die in a matter of months.

If Mr Brown was a patient in your present Health District, what services are available for the care of the terminally ill and could be taken into consideration in making decisions about his care?

What services and types of care are not available in your district? Does their absence present problems in caring for terminally ill patients like Mr Brown?

Mr Brown's pleural effusion was drained and the cytotoxic drug Bleomycin was instilled into the pleural space in order to slow down the probable reaccumulation of fluid. As a result Mr Brown was breathless on exertion rather than at rest as he had been. His pain was brought under control by his taking slow-release morphine tablets, and his constipation minimized by the use of a daily aperient.

Mr Brown's future medical care was planned to be shared between the hospital doctor and his general practitioner, and would be aimed towards controlling any symptoms he experienced. A community nurse visited Mr Brown and his family each week in order to assess their needs.

DISCUSSION AND FURTHER STUDY

Mr Brown's care in the final months of his life is going to be given principally by members of the primary health care team – his G.P. and community nurse in particular.

The organization of such care for the terminally ill can also be taken on by symptom control and support teams based in hospital or in hospices. These teams may offer support and care for patients and families in both hospital, hospice and community, wherever the patient's individual needs are best catered for.

1   The development of hospice care is outlined in Saunders 1986. You may like to follow up a number of the references she gives. This edition of the *Nursing Times* has a number of articles on care of the dying, including a study about the preferences of the terminally ill for home or hospital care.

2   Nursing research about caring for people with cancer is reported in the American nursing journals *Cancer Nursing* and *Oncology Nursing Forum*, and in nursing journals in the United Kingdom. One investigation into an attempt to devise a self-assessment tool for use with cancer patients is outlined in Holmes and Dickerson 1987.

3   Discussion about the relief of distressing symptoms in people with cancer raises the issue of euthanasia. *The Journal of Medical Ethics* has articles from time to time on this subject (e.g. Miller 1987).

4   You may be interested to explore further how nurses view the experience of nursing people with cancer. An investigation into this is reported in Wilkinson 1987.

REFERENCES TO VIGNETTE 3

KEY REFERENCES

Cahoon, M. C. 1982. *Cancer Nursing*. (Recent advances in nursing.) Churchill Livingstone, Edinburgh.

Tiffany, R. (ed.) 1978. *Oncology for Nurses and Health Care Professionals. Vol.I: Pathology, Diagnosis and Treatment*. Allen & Unwin, London.

Tiffany, R. (ed.) 1979. *Cancer Nursing. Radiotherapy*. Faber & Faber, London.

ADDITIONAL REFERENCES

Bond, S. 1983. Nurses' communication with cancer patients. In Wilson-Barnett, J. (ed.) *Nursing Research. Ten Studies in Patient Care. Developments in Nursing Research*, Vol.2. John Wiley & Sons, London.

Brown, M. et al. 1986. Lung cancer and dyspnea: the patient's perception. *Oncology Nursing Forum*, 13 (5), September/October, pp.19–24.

Foote, M. et al. (1986) Dyspnea: a distressing sensation in lung cancer. *Oncology Nursing Forum*. September/October, pp.25–31.

Hanks, G. W. 1983. Management of symptoms in advanced cancer. *Update*, 15 May, pp.1691–1702.

Holmes, S. 1986. Radiotherapy: minimising the side effects. *Professional Nurse*, I (10), July, pp.263–5.

Holmes, S. and Dickerson, J. 1987. The quality of life: design and evaluation of a self-assessment instrument for use with cancer patients. *International Journal of Nursing Studies*, 24 (I), pp.15–24.

Janes, G. 1986. Planning for terminal care. *Nursing Times*, 23 April, pp.24–7.

Miller, P. 1987. Death with dignity and the right to die: sometimes doctors have a duty to hasten death. *Journal of Medical Ethics*, 13 (2), June, pp.81–5.

Mumford, S. 1983. Nursing care study. Carcinoma of the bronchus. *Nursing Times*, 15 June, pp.48–50.

Saunders, C. 1986. The last refuge. *Nursing Times*, 22 October, pp.28–30.

Sofaer, B. 1984. *Pain: A Handbook for Nurses*. Lippincott Nursing Series. Harper & Row, London.

Taylor, A. 1983. An alternative to surgery. *Nursing Mirror*, 27 July, pp.29–32.

Walker, V. A. 1982. Skin care during radiotherapy. *Nursing Times*, 8 December, pp.2068–70.

Wilkinson, S. 1987. The reality of nursing cancer patients. *Lampada*, No.12, Summer. Pp.12–19.

Wilson-Barnett, J. 1979. *Stress in Hospital. Patients' Psychological Reactions to Illness and Health Care*. Churchill Livingstone, Edinburgh.

Yasko, J. M. 1982. *Care of the Client Receiving External Radiation Therapy*. Reston Publishing Inc., Virginia.

ANNE ELLIS

Anne is an elderly person who collapses at home after a stroke. She needs nutritional advice and follow-up in the community after her discharge.

The high proportion of elderly people in our society, together with, in its widest sense, the 'health problems' associated with the process of ageing, means that we, as nurses, need to be knowledgeable and skilful in our professional care of elderly people.

What experiences do you have of being with elderly people, other than those encountered in your nursing work?

What experiences concerning the nursing of elderly people come to mind? What have you learnt from those experiences?

CHECK ▶

Make sure you understand and investigate the following before completing the study questions of this vignette (see key references on page 120 for useful publications):

1 ▶   The process of ageing in physiological, psychological and social terms.

2 ▶   The constituents of a healthy diet for an elderly person.

3 ▶   The physical, psychological and social effect of cerebrovascular accidents for patients.

Anne Ellis, aged 81, lives in a terraced house near the railway station in Manchester. She was widowed thirteen years ago. Her only relative is a niece who lives in Liverpool. Mrs Ellis lives frugally on her state pension and a very small widow's pension. She lives an independent life and manages her domestic activities herself. Her pride and joy are her two cats.

One morning, during a very cold period of winter weather, Mrs Ellis collapses in her kitchen whilst washing up her breakfast crockery. She finds it impossible to get back on to her feet again and lies on the floor until her neighbour, Mrs Neve, comes in the back door on her usual evening visit with the newspaper and some milk.

Mrs Neve, on finding that Mrs Ellis is disorientated and looks as though she has experienced a stroke, enlists the help of her husband who telephones Mrs Ellis' GP. Together they lift Mrs Ellis on to the settee in the living room and wrap her in an eiderdown, since her body feels cold and they know that hypothermia is a problem for elderly people in this sort of situation.

Mrs Neve and her husband are quite right to be concerned about hypothermia in elderly people.

Think about the advice that you could offer to elderly people themselves, and to their neighbours and relatives, in order to minimize the avoidable causes of hypothermia. (See Roper et al 1985, Ch.13., Green 1986; Saddington 1983; Hillman 1987.)

After the GP's visit Mrs Ellis is admitted to her local community hospital for observation and assessment. She arrives there at 9 p.m., and is fully conscious and upset about 'being a nuisance'.

Assuming you have only the background information given so far, write an outline of the essential features in this patient's history that you would focus on when conducting an initial nursing assessment that evening.

You probably identified that whilst Mrs Ellis was hypothermic, and probably disorientated and frightened by her experience, an initial nursing assessment would need to take into account, at the very least, to what extent she was able to be independent in the activities of living, and consequently the sort of nursing assistance she would need initially.

Think again about what you would assess and draw up some initial ideas about what should be written on her care plan for use overnight.

For two priority areas of care, see Carr and Shepherd 1979, Newman 1985 (positioning a stroke patient); Anthony 1987 (pressure area care).

During the following morning, after Mrs Ellis has rested overnight, she is reassessed. Her medical assessment reveals that she has experienced a right-sided cerebrovascular accident (C.V.A.) resulting in left-sided hemiplegia, and that she is mildly anaemic, as her haemoglobin level is 10.0 grams per 100 mls of blood.

Her nursing assessment, using Roper's framework, is summarized and outlined below:

◊ Left-sided hemiplegia. Is fully conscious and seems aware of the weakness on her left side when her attention is drawn to it.

◊ Some slight difficulty with articulation when trying to speak, but was able to explain what happened to her yesterday. She thinks she 'blacked out for a while'. Neighbour, Mrs Neve, is best friend, niece visits monthly.

◊   Ate porridge, marmalade and bread and two cups of tea without help. Is aware that she dribbled. Feels thirsty. ? underweight, but says she has always been thin.

◊   Has passed urine since admission, was incontinent on admission and since. Used a bedpan successfully during this assessment and will need to be given opportunity to void two hourly until she settles and can summon a nurse. No history of constipation, bowels were opened yesterday.

◊   Personal level of hygiene and grooming very good. Dentures well fitting.

◊   Mildly hypothermic on admission, temperature at 6 a.m. 37°.

◊   Left hemiplegia, normally mobility is good. Walks half a mile to shops.

◊   Does housework and shopping. Watches TV, reads, knits, looks after cats.

◊   Well-groomed person. Wishes to wear her own nightclothes when neighbour brings them in. Self-sufficient and capable, and proud of her continuing independence despite her age.

◊   Rested well overnight. Sleeps well at home.

◊   Vital signs: B.P. $\frac{155}{75}$; pulse 80 beats per minute.

Mrs Ellis has three principal problems:

1   her left-sided paralysis;
2   some lack of awareness and inability to control micturition;
3   some dysarthria.

What nursing will be planned to maximize the possibility of her overcoming these problems?
(See Cole 1986 on speech difficulties, and Norton 1984 on incontinence.)

Two weeks later Mrs Ellis is again reassessed:

◊   Speech very little affected by stroke now.

◊   Eating and drinking without assistance. Says she eats anything and is interested in 'eating better' from now on.

◊   No incontinence. Can manage to sit on toilet on her own by using side rails. Bowel movements normal.

◊   Needs no assistance when washing at sink provided she has chair to sit on and can use taps to help her to stand up. Is able to dress herself.

◊　　Is walking with tripod. Finds it tiring, and at present likes to have someone nearby 'just in case'.

◊　　Has been reading and watching TV – thinks she may take up tapestry work.

◊　　Hair washed and set by hospital hairdresser, puts hair rollers in at night. Wears day clothes all day.

After her discharge, Mrs Ellis plans to spend three weeks at her niece's home in Liverpool. She will then be collected by Mr and Mrs Neve (her neighbours) and taken to her home.

Taking into account Mrs Ellis' most recent assessment, outline her plan of care for the following week until her discharge.

Mrs Ellis would like to 'eat better' in the future. Her usual day's menu is as follows:

Breakfast	2 cups of tea with sugar white bread or toast with marmalade and butter
Midmorning	cup of tea with sweet biscuits
Lunch	sliced cold meat from butcher or from a tin, or a pork pie pickle, pickled onions cup of tea
Supper	fish and chips twice a week via Mrs Neve pie or pastry (ready made) with mashed potato (sometimes made with dried potato power) instant gravy granules, tinned peas or carrots white bread and butter tinned rice pudding or ice-cream

Mrs Ellis says she 'can't be bothered' to spend lots of time in food preparation and does not know about what sorts of food would provide a more 'healthy' way of eating.

What alterations in Mrs Ellis' eating habits do you feel are necessary? Explore why such changes would be beneficial.

What will influence Mrs Ellis' implementation of the alterations in her diet that you might propose?

Mrs Ellis is willing to change her eating habits in order to improve her health. Elderly people, sometimes contrary to expectations, are known to be willing to change their eating patterns, and a study by Bilderbeck *et al* (1981) outlines the food changes made by one group of elderly people.

Mrs Ellis will eventually be back in her own home and, until she feels so unwell as to need help from her GP, it is unlikely that she will be supported by any healthcare professionals. There is, however, a body of opinion which favours more active surveillance of the elderly by considering the social, environmental and psychological problems which, if left unchecked, can result in ill health. Potentially the community nurse and the health visitor have key roles in this sort of preventative work. (For further discussion of this topic, see Luker 1983, Day 1986, Stanton 1987 and Phillipson and Strang 1986a, b.)

DISCUSSION AND FURTHER STUDY

Mrs Ellis has managed to maintain her independence. Despite her vulnerability, her need to return to her own home has been respected and fostered by those who came into contact with her in hospital and those family members and friends who support her.

She intends to change some of her eating habits but does not wish to have the services of meals-on-wheels or a home help at present.

1 An interesting study about the nutrition of the elderly and the potential role of the meals-on-wheels service in improving it is described in Davies 1981. In addition, consider the impact the door-to-door milkman can have on the nutrition of elderly people by means of the wide range of food other than milk that he sells.
2 What seem to be the key issues in the care of the elderly today? Consider the content of the nursing journals in your library to help you find some answers.

REFERENCES TO VIGNETTE 4

KEY REFERENCES

Jefferys, M. 1987. An ageing Britain – what is its future? *Geriatric Nursing and Home Care*. July, pp.19–24.

Redfern, S. J. 1986. *Nursing Elderly People*. Churchill Livingstone, London.

Roberts, A. 1987. Systems of Life. Nutrition and the elderly. *Nursing Times*. 24 June, pp.51–4, 1 July, pp.55–8, and 12 August, pp.51–4.

Webster, S. G. P. 1983a. A healthy appetite for life: 1. *Journal of District Nursing*, 1(8), February, pp.4–5, 8.

Webster, S. G. P. 1983b. A healthy appetite for life: 2. *Journal of District Nursing*, 1(9), March, pp.4–5, 30.

ADDITIONAL REFERENCES

Anthony, D. 1987. Pointers to good care. *Nursing Times*, 26 August, pp.27, 29–30.

Bilderbeck, N. et al. 1981. Changing food habits among 100 elderly men and women in the United Kingdom. *Journal of Human Nutrition*, 35 (6), December, pp.448–55.

Carr, J. and Shepherd, R.1979. *Early Care of the Stroke Patient*. William Heinemann Medical Books, London.

Cole, J. 1986. A word in your ear. *Nursing Times*. 10 September, pp.53–4.

Davies, L. 1981. *Three Score Years . . . And Then?* William Heinemann Medical Books, London.

Day, L. 1986. Time to value the golden age. *Nursing Times*, 15 October, pp.67, 69.

Green, M. F. 1986. Maintaining body temperature. In Redfern, S. J. *Nursing Elderly People*. Churchill Livingstone, Edinburgh.

Hillman, H. 1987. The cold that kills. *Nursing Times*, 28 January, pp.19–20.

Luker, K. A. 1983. An evaluation of health visitors' visits to elderly women. In Wilson-Barnett, J. (ed.) *Nursing Research: 10 Studies in Patient Care*. John Wiley & Sons, Chichester.

Newman, D. 1985. Essential physical therapy for stroke patients. *Nursing Times*, 6 February, pp.16–18.

Norton, C. 1984. The promotion of continence. *Nursing Times*, 4 April. Supplement on incontinence, pp.4, 6, 8, 10.

Phillipson, C. and Strang, P. 1986a. Your role with the elderly. *Journal of District Nursing*, 4 (10), April, pp.11–12.

Phillipson, C. and Strang, P. 1986b. Your role with the elderly. *Journal of District Nursing*, 4(11), May, pp.13–14.

Roper, N., Logan, W. W. and Tierney, A. J. 1985. *The Elements of Nursing*, 2nd edn. Churchill Livingstone, Edinburgh.

Saddington, N. 1983. Winter of discontent? *Nursing Times*, 26 October, pp.10–11.

Stanton, A. 1987. Happy birthday. *Nursing Times*. Community Outlook, 11 March.

ROSA FRENCH

Rosa has rheumatoid arthritis and is admitted to hospital for respite care.

Some people live with pain and illness as a constant companion. They have to learn to adapt their lives so that they can cope more readily with the daily activities which many of us take for granted. Rheumatoid arthritis is a disease which can cause such deformity of joints that apparently simple tasks like unscrewing a jar top, creaming butter and sugar, undoing a button, sitting up and sitting down can become a major effort.

CHECK ▶

Before completing the study questions in this vignette make sure that you understand the following (see key references, page 126, for useful texts):

1 ▶ The anatomy and physiology of synovial joints;

2 ▶ The abnormal physiology of rheumatoid arthritis;

3 ▶ The abnormal physiology of osteo-arthrosis (arthritis).

Mrs Rosa French is a 56-year-old lady who has had rheumatoid arthritis for about twelve years. For the last two to three years she has been really incapacitated and has had to live on the ground floor of her house. She can't walk up the stairs as her knees are deformed and very painful. Her hands are in a similar condition and she is unable to cope with fine movements.

She has been admitted to a hospital for assessment while her husband, who is her chief carer, takes a holiday.

What points would you consider when taking a nursing history?

What specific questions do you think you may ask?

One useful, all-encompassing question here is 'how do you spend your day at home?' This will give you a clear idea about how she copes, how much her husband has to do for her, and what strategies she has developed for making herself comfortable and for coping with life as effectively as she possibly can.

Rosa has brought her own chair into hospital with her and a support pillow for use in bed. She has splints which she wears on her hands overnight. These 'rest' splints are made of light-weight plastic and are worn during periods of repose to prevent deformity.

During her conversation with you, Rosa also mentions that she takes honey three times a day and she feels that this must be good for her arthritis and eases the pain.

You feel certain that there is no scientific reason to suppose that honey is effective in the treatment of rheumatoid arthritis or a relief of its symptoms. What do you think you should say to Rosa at this point?

In a sense this is an ethical dilemma in that you may feel that you should tell Rosa the truth, but on the other hand you may decide that as it's not doing her any harm and she believes in it she may well continue to take it. This is probably the kindest, and most sensible, solution.

Rosa tends to talk about her 'rheumatism'. What does she mean by this? What, for instance, is the difference between rheumatoid arthritis, from which Rosa suffers, and osteo-arthrosis or, if you prefer, osteo-arthritis? You may find it useful to draw up comparative lists.

The term rheumatism is really a lay term, a 'catch all' phrase which refers to all joint disease. Osteo-arthrosis is a degenerative disease which is why some experts in this field prefer to use this term rather than osteo-arthritis. The latter term suggests inflammation which is not present in this disease.

Rheumatoid arthritis, however, is a systemic, inflammatory disease and your reading will have shown you that its effects may be far reaching and not localized solely to the joints.

On her first night in hospital, it takes hours for you to settle Rosa comfortably. She clearly likes her pillow in a certain position, her joints rested in a very particular way, and is very specific about the order in which she should take her tablets. You have other patients to see to and know you'll be off duty late. You're very tired and know that you're on an early shift the next day.

How do you think you would cope in this situation?

This is a difficult problem, and one that you may have met before. It's quite interesting to ask yourself why this occurred and it is possible that inadequate history taking had led to not enough time being allowed to settle Rosa down for the night. It is probably best to be open with Rosa, and say that you had not realized quite how much time you would need to settle her and perhaps she would rather wait for the night staff who can help as soon as they have had their report. It may be that you could start by helping Rosa with her teeth and her mouth care, or apply her splints before actually trying to move her to settle down. Whatever you decide to do, honesty is probably the best policy and you can say to her that you will reassess the situation and record on her care plan specifically how she likes to be positioned at night and how long this may need.

In the past Rosa has been treated with drug therapy for her rheumatoid arthritis. The aim of drug therapy in this disease is to suppress the symptoms and to modify the progress of the disease. Symptom suppression is usually approached by use of anti-inflammatory drugs and Rosa has in the past taken aspirin; now she is taking Ibuprofen. The drug which Rosa takes to modify the disease is Salazopyrin, an immuno-suppressant drug. It is reported in the *Journal of District Nursing* February 1987 that this drug is now thought to cause macrocytic anaemia in which the red cells are larger, less efficient and fewer than normal as the drug interferes with folic acid. This anaemia is quickly reversed, however, by adding oral folic acid to the treatment.

Apart from drug therapy, in what other ways can Rosa's rheumatoid arthritis be treated?

The alternative to treatment by systemic means is to splint the deformed joints either internally or externally. Rosa has had one hip splinted internally in the past, in other words she has had a total hip replacement (see Watson and Royle 1987 and Hornsby 1985).

The management of somebody who has had a hip joint replaced is absolutely the same for both osteo-arthritis and rheumatoid arthritis.

Consider the nursing management of Rosa following her total hip replacement. What specific problems do you think nursing management may have been trying to prevent occurring?

Following any joint replacement the main potential problem which nursing management is trying to prevent is the dislocation of the joint. For this reason precautions will have been taken to ensure that Rosa did not cross her legs or move the affected hip which might cause the artificial ball and socket joint to come apart. If you can show a patient a prosthesis of the hip prior to surgery indicating the way in which the ball moves within the socket it becomes very clear to the patient why his or her movement is restricted during the first days after the operation.

It is crucial that someone like Rosa should not develop undue limb and joint stiffness or deformity as a result of post-operative immobility and active and passive movement of all other joints should be carried out.

People with rheumatoid arthritis are prone to very dry mouths and eyes. Mouth care to prevent inflammation and infection, and eye care to prevent drying up and crusting of the eyes, are of particular importance here.

When you talk to Rosa about her home life during the two weeks that she is in hospital it becomes obvious that the occupational therapist and social services have worked together to decide which particular equipment would benefit Rosa the most. She is fortunate, in that her husband has also been able to purchase various aids for her from the *Disabled Living Foundation*.

If you should ever get the opportunity to visit the Disabled Living Foundation in London, you will find it very interesting. If this isn't possible, then write to them and ask for information about the equipment and facilities which are available for the disabled. This will give you a clear idea of the problems which somebody with a crippling disease such as rheumatoid arthritis has to overcome.

It is not only sophisticated equipment which can help Rosa. The use of simple resourceful ideas, such as applying velcro to clothes instead of buttons so that she is more able to dress herself, and making a biscuit-based desert rather than using pastry so that she doesn't have to cream ingredients together, can be equally valuable.

Because Rosa has been ill for a long time, because she is in pain, and because she is probably the person who knows best how she can be made comfortable and how she can be helped, she may at times seem rather 'demanding'.

Look up any research or references that you can find regarding patients who are seen to be 'difficult' or 'not popular'. What conclusions do you draw from this about what makes a 'good' patient?

At the end of two weeks Rosa's husband, feeling much refreshed from his holiday, comes to collect her. He certainly looks well and younger than he did two weeks ago. You greet him and say, 'I'm sure Rosa is looking forward to seeing you.' His response is, 'I wish I could say the same. I just didn't want to come home. My Rosa's no longer the lady I married and looking after her has been really very difficult. I hadn't realized that until I had two weeks away from her.'

How would you respond to Mr French? This may be something that you would like to discuss with your colleagues. (See McFarlane 1985).

This is one of the many situations in which there is no right or wrong answer. All you can really do is acknowledge what the husband is saying and listen to him. Certainly it would be wrong to make any value judgement, and certainly the husband does have a difficult role to fulfil.

If you listen sensitively, and pick up on the cues which Rosa's husband may provide you with, it may be possible for you to identify what specific elements of the caring role are a problem to him. It may be, for instance, that he feels house-bound and misses his friends and his work. It may be that there is friction between Rosa and her husband because they are so much in each other's company for so much of the time. Another alternative may be that Rosa's husband misses taking the 'husband role'; he can no longer be the bread winner, he may miss coming home to a hot meal. Or perhaps he resents losing the sexual side of his marriage. These are all points to look for and it is possible that you could tentatively investigate the situation further by asking whether there is anyone who could help Rosa's husband in the caring role, or relieve him of his duties for one day a week for example. As it would seem that Rosa and her husband are well organized, it is very likely that he has been in touch with the pressure groups relating to this illness. There is a list of these in the back of Watson and Royle (1987) and Roper (1985), and the British Rheumatism and Arthritis Association will answer queries relating to all aspects of the disease and the help which may be given to those who care for people suffering from arthritis.

DISCUSSION AND FURTHER STUDY

In this vignette we've looked at the needs of a lady who is becoming increasingly disabled. We have considered her possible problems on her admission to hospital and have started to think about the needs that the main carer at home (in this case her husband) may experience.

In completing this vignette you might like to study further:

1 We met Rosa after she had had this disease for some years. Perhaps you would like to 'fill in' the story from the beginning. What do you think Rosa's initial symptoms were? How do you think she felt when she was first diagnosed?

2 In a situation like this, where you have one spouse caring for the other, where do you think the rights and duties of the individual lie? You may like to discuss this with your colleagues.

REFERENCES TO VIGNETTE 5

KEY REFERENCES

Dickinson, G..1985. Evaluation of an arthritis continuing education programme. *Journal of Continuing Education in Nursing* 16 (4), July/August, pp.127–31.

1987. Treating arthritis (drug treatment). *Journal of District Nursing*, February. Vol.5, No.8.

Roper, N., Logan, W. W. and Tierney, A. J. 1985. *The Elements of Nursing*, 2nd edition Churchill Livingstone, Edinburgh.

Scott, J. T. 1980. *Rheumatism: The Facts*. Oxford University Press, London.

Swinson, V. R. and Swinburne, W. R. 1980. *Rheumatology*. Hodder & Stoughton, London.

Watson, J. E. and Royle, J. R. 1987. *Watson's Medical-Surgical Nursing and Related Physiology*, 3rd edition. Baillière Tindall, London.

ADDITIONAL REFERENCES

Hornsby, V. 1985. Osteo-arthritis of the hip joint. *Nursing. The Add-on Journal of Clinical Nursing*, 2(48), December, pp.1318–20.

McFarlane, Ann. 1985. When givers prove unkind. *Nursing Mirror*, 161, 2 October, pp.36–7.

LYDIA FRANCIS

Lydia has multiple sclerosis and is cared for by her husband at home.

There are people who live a large part of their lives with illness, disease or disability as a constant companion. People with such problems cannot always cope with them in isolation but must rely on the support of relatives, friends and health workers to enable them to live life as fully as possible.

Do you know of anyone with such problems? Think about this person and any ways in which he or she may strive to prevent a disability from becoming a handicap.

CHECK ▶

In this vignette, we will be considering the needs of someone who is suffering from multiple sclerosis. Before you read on, ensure that you understand the following (see key references on page 132 for guidelines):

1 ▶   the structure of the spinal cord;

2 ▶   the ways in which multiple sclerosis may manifest itself;

3 ▶   the abnormal physiology which precipitates multiple sclerosis.

Lydia Francis is a 34-year-old nurse. She is currently unable to work as she is suffering from multiple sclerosis, which has restricted her mobility to the extent that she often needs to use a wheelchair in order to get around the house. She has an 8-year-old son, a 10-year-old daughter and her husband, Alan, is a fireman.

More than 50,000 people in Britain have multiple sclerosis, that is 1 in 1,200 of the population. Because there is no certainty about the cause of the disease there is no cure for it. There is also no active treatment, not least because every single case of multiple sclerosis is different. One person may be virtually unaffected while at the other end of the scale another person may become paralysed.

From your reading, you will have learned that multiple sclerosis is a disease which affects the central nervous system, that is the brain and the spinal cord. The disease attacks the myelin sheath, the layer of insulation which protects our nerve endings. The myelin is replaced by scar tissue – sclerosis. It is 'multiple' because the scars can occur anywhere, even in the brain itself. The damage to the myelin sheath means that the nerve impulses are prevented from reaching their destination, and various parts of the body stop working properly. This could lead to anything from temporary loss of sight, speech irregularities, incontinence or even paralysis. It would be wrong, however, to assume that multiple sclerosis always leads to rapid physical decline. Fewer than one person in ten will ever need to use a wheelchair. It does not affect intelligence, and it is not infectious, contagious or hereditary.

Lydia was first diagnosed as having multiple sclerosis when she was 26 years old, shortly after the birth of her son.

At this point you may like to consider the ways in which this disease may first have manifested itself. Consider also Lydia's and Alan's possible reactions to learning that she was suffering from multiple sclerosis. What will you tell them both.

There are usually at least two separate signs that someone has multiple sclerosis. Most often the first effect is on the optic nerve, and blurred vision occurs. Often, too, there are pins and needles in the arms or hands; add to that a bout of incontinence, and these are classic signs of multiple sclerosis.

Lydia will probably be worried that her disease will limit all areas of her life. Doctors often stress to a newly diagnosed patient that the disease may not be as damaging as they fear. It may never progress further than temporary paralysis of one hand. One feature of multiple sclerosis is that an inflammatory attack is followed by a period of remission, when the disease stops in its tracks for a varying length of time. It does recur, however.

Alan felt very bitter when the diagnosis was first made and his reaction was, understandably 'why us, why now, and what is going to happen in the future?' The most anyone can do for Alan at this time is listen to him. His thoughts may be totally for Lydia yet they equally may be centred upon his own needs. It would be wrong to consider that this is selfish of him and it is crucial that anyone in this position is given a chance to voice his personal fears.

So little is still known about the cause of multiple sclerosis that it would be difficult for anyone to give Alan factual information which would help him to come to terms with the situation. It is thought to be caused by a combination of viruses which attack before the age of fifteen and precipitate a susceptibility to multiple sclerosis. The first signs of the disease usually emerge at any time between the ages of twenty and forty.

In what ways might the role of individual family members have altered as a response to Lydia's illness? Consider here, too, the economical constraints that may be placed upon the family as a result of this long-term illness.

Lydia's aim is to live as independent a life as possible. Indeed, she has periods of remission when this is totally possible. However, she does have lapses where her gait becomes increasingly unsteady, her eyesight is bad, and incontinence is a problem. At times she suffers from irregularity of speech; her talking is slurred and she has difficulty in controlling the tone of her voice. In other words, there are periods when Lydia should not be left on her own.

When we consider that Alan's job is that of a fireman it becomes evident that he will probably have to alter his work pattern or even his job to accommodate Lydia's needs. The children, too, have to take on responsibilities greater than would normally be expected at their age.

There are many aids which Lydia may be able to use to help with walking, to make her more comfortable in bed, to act as protection during periods of incontinence, and to assist her with manual tasks if the hands are weak.

The Disabled Living Foundation will prove to be a useful resource if you wish to gain information about the aids and equipment which are available.

Financial help is available in the form of, for example, an attendance allowance if her husband has to give up his job to look after Lydia. Other allowances such as a telephone allowance may also be appropriate.

Next time you pass your local DHSS Office, call in to see what leaflets relating to available financial help you can find.

In an attempt to prevent further attacks, Lydia should be aware of the conditions which are known to stimulate an attack of multiple sclerosis. A hot bath can act as a trigger, pregnancy exacerbates the condition, and any infection, especially of the bladder, can cause a relapse. Doctors often advise patients to avoid stress and over-tiredness. A balanced diet is also part of the self-help advice.

The main treatment for multiple sclerosis is steroid therapy, which is often given routinely, when someone has a relapse, to reduce inflammation and swelling around the nerves. However, steroids do not have a marked effect on the progress of the disease, although there are now trials of immuno-suppressant drugs and the drug cyclosporin. Some sufferers have personal remedies. Sunflower oil, for example, is believed by many to alleviate the symptoms.

During the past eight years Lydia has been admitted to hospital twice. On each occasion it was so that she could be catheterized during a period of acute incontinence.

How would you assess Lydia on admission to hospital so that you can meet each of her individual needs? (See Roper 1985.)

If you have used Roper's work as a key reference, you have probably considered Lydia's individual needs in relation to each of the activities of living. It is important that people who cope with long-term disabilities at home should be able to adhere to their routine and use their own equipment as much as possible when they are in hospital. Throughout her illness it is possible that Lydia's self-image has been damaged, and not acknowledging her personal control of her illness will do nothing to raise her own self-esteem.

Lydia has had to give up her work as a result of her illness. She feels that she cannot be a proper mother to her children, and is aware that she cannot take part in a satisfying sexual relationship as often as her husband would like. She is an intelligent lady and her illness has in no way affected this. Here appearance is still very important to her.

Nursing care, therefore, must allow for Lydia to be involved in all the decisions made regarding her treatment and should be centred upon her wishes. If she wishes to wear her own clothes, to put on make-up and to have her hair washed regularly, then time should be made to give her help with this where necessary.

DISCUSSION AND FURTHER STUDY

We have briefly looked at some of the issues surrounding a disabled lady and her husband. The health caring professionals are not of prime importance in Lydia's care. It is Alan who has assumed that role. They need, too, advice and help from action groups. Perhaps you would like to contact one or two of the organizations below to see how they function and what facilities they provide.

1   The Multiple Sclerosis Society of Great Britain and Northern Ireland. There are 330 local branches throughout the country. Head Office is at 286, Munster Road, Fulham, London SW6.
2   Action for Research into Multiple Sclerosis (A.R.M.S.). This organization can be contacted through Research Unit, Central Middlesex Hospital, Acton Lane, London NW10.
3   The Disabled Living Foundation gives information and advice on aspects of disability. It holds displays and gives demonstrations of aids and gadgets.
4   Sexual Problems of the Disabled (S.P.O.D.). This organization, based in London, gives counselling on sexual problems.

REFERENCES TO VIGNETTE 6

KEY REFERENCES

Allen, S. 1987. Arms extended. *Nursing Times*. 28 October, 83 (83), p.44.

Capildeo, R. and Maxwell, 1982. *Progress in Rehabilitation: Multiple Sclerosis*.

Kohner, N. 1988. *Caring at Home*. King's Fund Centre, London.

Matthews, B. 1980. *Multiple Sclerosis: The Facts*. Oxford University Press, London.

Roper, N, Logan, W. W. and Tierney, A. J. 1985. *The Elements of Nursing*, 2nd edition. Churchill Livingstone, Edinburgh.

Watson, J. E. and Royle, J. R. 1987. *Watson's Medical-Surgical Nursing and Related Physiology*, 3rd edition. Baillière Tindall, London.

BIPTI GOPAL

Bipti is admitted to hospital with a ruptured appendix.

Becoming ill and needing help from health care professionals brings with it many worries about a person's future, about their ability to cope and the effect their illness will have on their family. This anxiety will be increased if the person is from an ethnic minority group, does not speak English, and experiences a lack of awareness or an unwillingness on the part of the health care professionals to make provision for their special needs.

Bring to mind the people from minority cultural and racial groups you have nursed.

What was the experience like for you?

What do you think the experience was like for these people?

CHECK ▶ Before completing the study questions in this vignette, investigate the way of life of some or all of the following cultural groups in British society:

(a)   people of Pakistani origin;
(b)   people of Indian origin;
(c)   people of Bangladeshi origin;
(d)   people of Afro-Caribbean origin.

(See key references on page 136 for some useful literature.)

Mrs Gopal was aware of the pain she felt over the whole of her abdomen, and the nausea too. She had prepared breakfast for her family and her daughter Karuna had taken the younger children off to school. They both went to the clothing factory, in which they worked, at the usual time.

Just before noon Mrs Gopal stood up in order to leave her sewing machine to go to the toilet and fainted. Karuna knew that her mother had not been feeling well but quickly realized that this was serious. On recovering consciousness Mrs Gopal continued to experience severe pain over the whole of her abdomen and insisted on lying on the floor and not moving. The manager rang for an ambulance and Mrs Gopal was persuaded to allow herself to be taken to hospital.

On arrival in the accident and emergency department, Mrs Gopal was transferred to an examination trolley in a curtained cubicle. Sister assessed the situation and established what symptoms she was experiencing by using Mrs Gopal's daughter, Karuna, as an interpreter.

If you were the nurse asked by Sister to 'get this patient ready for the doctor', what would you do?

How would your first observations that the person is a woman, of probably Asian origin, unable to speak English, in pain, and wearing a sari and blouse, influence your actions? (See Henley 1980, *Nursing Times* 1981.)

Mrs Gopal is examined by Dr Joyce Green at Sister's request. Sister enables Karuna to contact her father to ask him to come straight to the hospital as Mrs Gopal may need surgery urgently and may need to consult him before agreeing to undergo surgery and signing a consent form.

It is thought that Mrs Gopal has a perforated appendix and so she is prepared for surgery.

How would you prepare a patient for an emergency appendicectomy?

How will meeting the individual needs of this person, Mrs Gopal, who does not speak English and is a Hindu, alter the usual format of routine pre-operative care for this form of surgery?

Following appendicectomy, in which it was found that the appendix was very inflamed and had ruptured, Mrs Gopal returns to a surgical ward to recover from the anaesthetic and the surgery. She has a naso-gastric tube, intravenous fluids and a wound drain. Her care includes the administration of intravenous fluids and antibiotics.

What nursing will be planned for Mrs Gopal:
(a)   on her return to the ward?
(b)   for her first and second post-operative days?
(c)   in what way can her care be individualized and take into account that she is unable to speak English and observes the Hindu religion?

(See Ellison Nash 1980, Royal Marsden Hospital 1984)

Four days after admission Mrs Gopal is making a good recovery. She is able to walk around with minimal discomfort, her temperature is normal, she is drinking about 2½ litres of fluid in 24 hours. She has begun eating again and her family bring food into hospital for her.

Investigate the dietary and meal time requirements of people who are of the Hindu religion.

Mrs Gopal spends much of the day on her own, because although many of her fellow patients acknowledge her with a smile they do not include her in their socializing. However, during the day she has many visitors. She prefers to stay on or near her bed in a bay occupied by women, as other parts of the ward accommodate male patients.

How would you set about planning Mrs Gopal's discharge from hospital?

DISCUSSION AND FURTHER STUDY

Patients have individual needs and nurses try to meet those needs. Assessing and meeting the needs of Mrs Gopal is complicated by the nurses' inability to speak her language. However, Mrs Gopal's family anticipate the problems that might arise from this and ensure that they communicate Mrs Gopal's needs to the staff and vice versa.

1 Investigate the provision made by your health district to meet the special needs of patients from ethnic minority groups.
2 One of the most important needs of a patient from a different culture who is unable to speak fluent English is for the nurse or other health care professional to continue to acknowledge and communicate with him or her.

Think about the implications for your practice of the following suggestions made by Mares *et al.* (1985) of practical ways of overcoming communication problems with patients of minority cultural and racial origins.

(*a*)   Allow more time than you would normally.
(*b*)   Give plenty of non-verbal reassurance by means of smiling, touching where appropriate, giving gestures of encouragement, and have a sympathetic manner.
(*c*)   Try to communicate information about what is going to happen; never maintain total silence or give the impression of ignoring the patient.
(*d*)   Get the patient's name right and try to pronounce it correctly.
(*e*)   Keep comprehensive written records of information about the patient.
(*f*)   Try to ensure that the patient sees the same staff members as far as possible.
(*g*)   Try to find out specific worries and fears that the patient may have.
(*h*)   Write down important information for the patient to take away with them on discharge.

REFERENCES FOR VIGNETTE 7

KEY REFERENCES

Dobson, S. 1983. Bringing culture into care. *Nursing Times*, 9 February, pp.53, 56–7.

McGilloway, O. and Myco, F. (eds) 1985. *Nursing and Spiritual Care*. Harper & Row, London.

Mares, P., Henley, A., and Baxter, C. 1985. *Health Care in Multiracial Britain*. Health Education Council/National Extension College.

Sampson, C. 1982. *The Neglected Ethic: Religious and Cultural Factors in the Care of Patients*. McGraw-Hill, Maidenhead.

Webb, P. 1982. The clash of cultures – health care. *Nursing*, 2 (1), May, pp.20–21.

ADDITIONAL REFERENCES

Ellison Nash, D. F. 1980. *The Principles and Practice of Surgery for Nurses and Allied Professions*, 7th edition. Edward Arnold, London.

Henley, A. 1979. *Asian Patients in Hospital and at Home*. King Edward's Hospital Fund for London. Distributed by Pitman Medical Publishing Co., Tunbridge Wells. For an article based on this book, see *Nursing Times Chatsheet: Community Outlook*. July 1981, pp.239–41.

Henley, A. 1980. Practical care of Asian patients. *Nursing*, 16 August, pp.683–6.

Royal Marsden Hospital. 1984. *Manual of Clinical Nursing Policies and Procedures*. Lippincott Nursing Series, Harper & Row, London.

PETER GRAY

Peter has AIDS and is admitted to hospital.

Caring for people with Acquired Immune Deficiency Syndrome, AIDS, in hospital or in the community is a challenge for us as nurses. We need to help people with the distressing symptoms of a fatal illness, one which carries with it such stigma that the person is sometimes ostracized by others. It is also a challenge because it may be the case that the care we give may be affected by our own prejudices and fears about the disease.

Have you helped nurse a person with AIDS in hospital or in the community?

What did you learn from this experience?

If you have not had this experience, try writing down your immediate concerns about nursing people with AIDS.

CHECK ▶

Make sure you understand and investigate the following before completing the study questions in this vignette (see key references on page 141 for helpful literature):

1 ▶ The concept of immunity and the process of antibody formation.

2 ▶ The relationship between Human Immunodeficiency Virus, HIV, and Acquired Immune Deficiency Syndrome, AIDS, or AIDS-Related Complex, ARC. (The Royal College of Nursing will supply a bibliography about this subject if requested.)

3 ▶ The ways in which a person can be infected by HIV.

Peter Gray is twenty-six, and a teacher, but he has been too unwell to work for the past six months. He is now a patient on a general medical ward and was admitted with AIDS, with the key problems of pneumonia and dehydration. Until his admission he had been cared for at home by John. But as Peter became increasingly more breathless and had pain, cough and fever, both agreed with their GP that Peter needed to be admitted to hospital.

Given the information you have so far, what initial care will Peter need on admission?

Peter is assessed when his pain has been relieved and he feels less breathless. His assessment takes into account the framework developed by Pratt (1986). Pratt outlines what he terms 'stragetic nursing care' for patients with HIV-related illness. He adapts some of the ideas of Virginia Henderson and of Nancy Roper, and formulates his own fifteen 'requisites for health' which are used as a basis for assessing patients' needs. They are as follows:

1   the need for adequate respiration;
2   the need for adequate hydration;
3   the need for adequate nutrition;
4   the need for urinary and faecal elimination;
5   the need to control body temperature;
6   the need for movement and mobilization;
7   the need for a safe environment;
8   the need for personal cleansing and dressing;
9   the need for expression and communication;
10 the need for working and playing;
11 the need for adequate rest and sleep;
12 the need to maintain psychological equilibrium*
13 the need to worship according to his own faith;
14 the need to express sexuality;
15 needs associated with dying.

*For number 12, 'the need to maintain psychological equilibrium', the nurse assesses to what extent the patient is anxious, how well he is coping, his degree of social isolation, his self esteem and whether he is depressed.

What do you think of Pratt's ideas? Would you find such a framework helpful in assessing patients?

Peter's initial nursing assessment shows that his principal needs are:
1   to breathe normally, without effort or pain;
2   to get sufficient sleep and rest so that he feels refreshed;
3   to stop feeling nauseated, so that he can eat and regain some weight, and to be able to drink to overcome the problems of dehydration, dry skin and mouth;
4   to feel well again, to feel sexually attractive and desirable, and to feel hopeful about the future.

Outline some nursing activities which could be planned to meet Peter's needs, 1, 2 and 3.

How can his needs outlined in 4 be met? What resources are available to meet them?

Peter is being nursed in a four-bedded bay opposite the nurses' station. He feels reassured by the presence of staff, although he finds that it can be rather noisy at times. His fellow patients are Graham Blount with sickle cell crisis, and Edward Ellison who is unconscious following a cerebrovascular accident.

Peter's white blood cell count is below normal, though not excessively so, but he is very vulnerable to infection. A vital part of his care is to maintain his personal hygiene, particularly his oral hygiene, and to prevent cross-infection from staff members, from patients and the hospital environment generally. Though prevention of cross-infection is an essential part of nursing practice, patients who are particularly vulnerable, like Peter, require that staff be constantly vigilant.

The Human Immunodeficiency Virus, HIV, is transmitted sexually, by inoculation into the bloodstream, and perinatally. What precautions need to be taken by hospital staff who come into contact with Peter to prevent them being affected by the virus?

Consider the current DHSS guidelines and those produced by the Royal College of Nursing. Compare the guidelines of these organizations with those of your own Health Authority. (See Glenister 1986, Elliot 1987.)

Peter's pneumonia is caused by the micro-organism *pneumocystis carinii* and so he is given intravenous co-trimoxazole, an antibiotic. The oxygen levels in his blood are abnormal and he is given continuous oxygen therapy to help to correct this.

What are the unwanted effects of this antibiotic and what observations will you make to detect these?

What care will Peter need whilst having oxygen therapy?

Peter has not seen his parents for a couple of years. They know where he lives and his telephone number, but they do not contact him even on such occasions as his birthday or at Christmas. This is principally because they feel unable to accept him and his homosexuality. His sister Andrea does see him, and rings him at least once a month. She had been unaware that he was HIV positive initially, but Peter explained the situation to her when he experienced his first bout of feeling ill, again with a chest infection, six months ago.

Nursing patients requires us to take into account fundamental ethical principles such as respect for persons, and to be concerned with patients' rights to privacy, to being given information about themselves, and being given the opportunity to exercise choice.

Think through how you would deal with the following situations which arise whilst nursing Peter.

(a)   Another patient asks you what is wrong with the man in bed 15, Peter, and asks 'Is it catching?'.

(b)   Peter's parents ring up and ask how he is. In the course of the conversation they ask 'What actually is wrong with our Peter?'.

(c)   A nurse from an agency is sent to the ward by Nursing Administration as the nursing team has two members of staff away ill. The agency nurse refuses to help in any way with the care of Peter. (See Dimond 1987).

Much of Peter's personal care over the weekend is given by John who spends most of the day in the ward. Peter and John are visited and gain support from a volunteer, Michael, from the Terence Higgins Trust. Together Peter and John both face the strong possibility of dying whilst young. After Peter's death, John, who is HIV positive, will have to face bouts of ill health without the support of Peter and the likelihood of his own untimely death. (See Wells 1987 regarding nursing care and support in this situation).

Five days later Peter's temperature is back to normal, he no longer needs continuous oxygen and he is beginning to feel able to face food again.

How would you set about planning for Peter's discharge home?

What community care and support can be offered to Peter and John?

DISCUSSION AND FURTHER STUDY

Nursing people with AIDS requires us as nurses to practise skilfully to prevent infection being transmitted from patient to nurse, and from nurse to patient. It requires us to promote the comfort and dignity of the person and to give support and help to enable him to face this terminal illness.

1   Try to assess critically the way in which people with AIDS are presented in the media. What attitudes towards them underlie the presentation of the story or report? Is the factual basis of the story accurate or inaccurate given present knowledge about the illness and its transmission?

2   Critically assess the Government's publicity campaigns directed towards the general public by means of leaflets, television, radio and newspaper advertisements. What messages about this disease are being transmitted?

3   Compare and contrast the policies and procedures of your hospital or health authority concerning patients with HIV and those with hepatitis B.

REFERENCES TO VIGNETTE 8

KEY REFERENCES

Pratt, R. J. 1986. *AIDS: A Stragegy for Nursing Care*. Edward Arnold, London.

Schober, P. 1987. AIDS: Facing the facts. *Nursing Times*, 4 March, pp.28–31.

Wells, N. 1986. *The AIDS Virus*. Office of Health Economics, London.

ADDITIONAL REFERENCES

Dimond, B. 1987. In case of AIDS. *Nursing Times*, 3 June, pp.27–9.

Elliot, J. 1987. ABC of AIDS: Nursing care. *British Medical Journal*, 295, 11 July, pp.104–6.

Glenister, H. M. 1986. AIDS and HTLV-III infection. *Nursing*, Vol.3, No.6, June, pp.229–31.

Wells, R. 1987. AIDS – a perspective of care. *International Nursing Review*, 34 (4), May/June, pp.64–6.

GEOFF LANE AND PERCY KNOWLES

Geoff and Percy are both admitted to hospital and undergo lower limb amputation.

The loss of a limb, for whatever reason, is possibly one of the most devastating events that can occur in anyone's life. Whether or not the pre-disposing factors which necessitate amputation can be deemed to be 'self-inflicted' may possibly influence the individual's adaptation processes following surgery.

Do you know of anyone who has had a limb amputated?

Why was this done?

How does he/she cope now?

CHECK ▶

Make sure you understand and investigate the following before completing the sudy questions:

1 ▶ Arterial circulation.

2 ▶ Factors which precipitate ischæmia.

(See key references page 146 for literature.)

Geoff Lane and Percy Knowles are patients on a ward where people are treated for vascular disorders. They have each had a right above-knee amputation. Geoff Lane's amputation was performed following an accident in which he, as a commuter, trapped his leg between train and platform on his way home from work. Percy's amputation was necessitated by peripheral vascular disease.

Before continuing, make sure you can answer the following questions:

1 Why may trauma necessitate amputation?
2 Why does peripheral vascular disease precipitate amputation?
(See Baum 1985).

Trauma can lead to massive necrosis of the muscle, and products of this dead muscle may be absorbed into the system causing toxaemia. It is necessary, therefore, to amputate in order to bring about what should be a dramatic improvement to the general condition.

Peripheral vascular disease will eventually lead to ischæmia. This in turn causes death of the tissue which then becomes infected gangrene. The resultant condition is extremely, persistently painful.

Percy Knowles has been a smoker for over fifty years. He is now sixty-nine years old. Cigarette smoking leads to the constriction of blood vessels. He has experienced pain for some months now. He cannot use his right leg to walk about and he is exhausted due to the lack of rest and sleep.

Geoff is thirty-five years old and works in City bank. He has a young family and has always enjoyed joining in with their weekend activities such as tennis, football and swimming.

Contrast the possible fears/needs/and reactions of the two men immediately post-operatively. (See Kelly 1985.)

Each of these men has had an operation which has changed his life dramatically. One will have had a chance to adjust himself gradually to the idea, the other will not. Each, at some point, may well experience grief for the person that he once was.

Percy possibly approached the operation with mixed feelings. The fact that he has been in pain for some time and unable to walk anyway may have made him feel more positive about having his leg amputated. Post-operatively, when the realization of the finality of the procedure hits him, he may well feel angry. There may be fear, too, centred around such questions as 'How will I manage?' 'Will the other leg go the same way?' If he is aware and accepts that smoking is very possibly the cause of the peripheral vascular disease, Percy Knowles may well also feel guilty and act defensively.

Geoff Lane's reactions may be similar although they may be ordered somewhat differently.

Have you ever nursed anyone who has been injured in an accident?

How did he/she react?

Very often, following a major accident, people are really unaware of what has happened. They may have been told what has occurred and what injuries they have sustained, but the reality of this does not always make a full, immediate impact. There is an awareness of pain, discomfort and a gratitude for anything which is done to relieve it. There is often consolation in the nearness of relatives and friends and a gratitude for their presence.

How often do you hear people say 'He's so brave and cheerful, you wouldn't believe what he's been though!'. The truth is that the patient probably doesn't believe it either.

It may be some time, then, before Geoff Lane admits his predicament to himself. He may even deny it until he is discharged home and becomes aware that some things in his life have changed for ever, not the least of which may be his own self-image.

Geoff, too, may feel guilty. Although his accident happened very quickly and had not in any way been foreseen, he may well think, 'If only I'd done something differently, none of this would have happened'.

Do you feel that either Geoff or Percy is more deserving of care?

Discuss this with your colleagues.

In the immediate post-operative period, the care of both Geoff and Percy will be aimed at rehabilitating them as soon as possible.

How do you think this could be achieved?

Try to identify the aims of care by yourself at this point.

Care will be aimed at:

1   monitoring general well being;
2   caring for the stump;
3   monitoring personal safety;
4   detecting pain and depression;
5   keeping the patient nourished;
6   exercising the whole body.

What nursing care would you implement to meet these aims?

Watson & Royle (1987) is particularly helpful here.

Both Percy and Geoff get up out of bed as soon as possible, although each needs help as balance is obviously difficult to maintain.

Each is taught to use crutches. Percy finds this difficult as his arms were considerably weakened during the period of his illness prior to surgery when he was confined to a chair for some weeks. Geoff finds it easier to use crutches but is loath to do so as he wants to wait until he has his artificial limb and will, as he says, 'at least look like a complete man when I stand up'. He finds it hard to accept that this will not happen for six weeks as the stump will not have shrunk to its final size until then, so there is little point in measuring for an artificial prosthesis.

Arrangements are made to discharge Geoff. He is told that when he goes to be measured for his permanent prosthesis he will probably have a temporary one fitted whilst the other is being made. He puts up much resistance to going home although he says he wants to be there. His objections are 'What will the children think of me?' 'How will I manage the stairs?' 'Why can't I stay here to practise walking?'

How will you respond to these questions?

Percy is more willing to go home. He wishes to use a wheelchair, as he did before the amputation, and says he can manage just as well as he did before in his ground floor flat.

Do you think he should be persuaded to use crutches, and have a prosthesis fitted against his wishes?

There is no right or wrong answer to this, but you may like to discuss the matter with colleagues.

DISCUSSION AND FURTHER STUDY

We have briefly looked at the needs of two gentlemen who have circulatory problems for very different reasons. You may have felt it was more of a tragedy for the younger one to have to cope with such a trauma, but it is worth considering that sometimes it is more difficult to adapt to new situations as we get older.

In completing this vignette, you may like to go on to consider the following.

1   Despite all that has happened to him, Percy continues to smoke heavily. Should you try to prevent this? If so how? You may like to further this discussion by considering whether people have the right to abuse their own bodies.

2   Where is your local limb-fitting centre?

What facilities does your local health authority use to help amputees in the process of rehabilitation?

REFERENCES TO VIGNETTE 9

KEY REFERENCES

Baum, P. 1985. Heed the early warning signs of peripheral vascular disease. *Nursing*, 15(3), March, pp.50–57.

Elwes, L. and Simnett, J. 1985. *Promoting Health. A Practical Guide to Health Education.* John Wiley & Sons, London.

Horton, R. E. 1980. *Vascular Surgery.* Hodder & Stoughton, London.

Kelly, M. D. 1985. Loss and grief reactions as responses to surgery. *Journal of Advanced Nursing*, 10(6), November, pp.17–25.

Watson, J. E. and Royle, J. R. 1987. *Watson's Medical-Surgical Nursing and Related Physiology*, 3rd edition. Baillière Tindall, London.

CHARLES LEWIS

Charles is killed in a road traffic accident on his way home from work.

There can be very few nurses who, at some time in their careers, have not felt inadequate. Supporting the bereaved in the event of a sudden death is an example of one such occasion.

Can you recall an instance when you were present at the time of a sudden death?

How did you feel?

What support did you feel you could give to the bereaved relatives or friends?

CHECK ▶

Before completing the study questions in this vignette, make sure you investigate and understand the following:

1 ▶   The grieving process.

2 ▶   The current extent of the drink-driving problem both locally and nationally.
(See key references on page 150. Also, reports of fatal accidents or summaries of local/ national accident figures in newspapers, journals and magazines can prove helpful.)

One evening, when you are working as a student in an accident and emergency department, two patients are admitted. One is a 30-year-old gentleman named Charles Lewis. He was knocked down by a car on a zebra crossing while he was on his way home from work, and has received severe head injuries. The other patient has a fractured tibia and fibula. He is the driver of the car, who was returning home from an office party when the accident occurred.

What is the legally acceptable amount of alcohol for drivers to have within their blood?

You can use your local police station as a resource here, or information centres such as the Alcohol Studies Centre. The DHSS publication: *Drug Misuse – a basic briefing* (February 1985) contains a section on alcohol in which the legal status of the substance is discussed.

If you have been successful in your literature search, you will know that it is an offence to drive whilst unfit to do so because of drink or with more than 80mg of alcohol in every 100ml of blood.

Charles's wife, Wendy, arrives in the department. Shortly after this, Charles dies.

What might be Wendy's initial reaction to this horrific event? (See Chaney 1980, ch.2.)

In this chapter, (see reference above) Dr Kubler-Ross describes the first stage of grief as being a state of shock and denial. Murray Parkes 1980 suggests that relatives in the event of a sudden death sense a greater numbness than those who have had a chance to anticipate the bereavement. They have had no time to process and incorporate what is happening, no time for reminiscing, no time to work out unfinished business.

Wendy Lewis' denial, therefore, may be totally adamant and take the form of 'No, he can't be dead, I've just bought his Christmas present (he's in the middle of decorating the house, I can't afford to pay the mortgage on my own' etc.)'. Yet, whatever her immediate reaction, it is unlikely that she will have appreciated the true reality of the situation.

How can you help Wendy at this time?

How may you feel?

It seems almost arrogant to assume that there is anything which anyone can do to help this lady at a time of such immense sorrow. The only resources available are, perhaps, time and the presence of a listening, sympathetic ear.

Nursing and other health care staff may well feel totally inadequate at this time, guilty because they feel they cannot offer any constructive help, and angry because this was a potentially preventable death. The presence of the car driver within the department might exacerbate this anger.

Wendy may, herself, demonstrate uncontrollable anger at this time. She could well experience utter and bitter resentment as a reaction to the situation in which she finds herself. It is possible that her anger will be directed at the car driver (though if the situation is well managed, Wendy will not even be aware that he's in the department). It is equally possible that the anger will be directed towards the very staff who are trying to help her.

Has it ever happened to you that a patient seemed to be irrationally cross with you?

When this happens, there is little you can do other than to accept the emotion for what it is – a response to circumstances rather than to you personally.

Using the book by Wright (1986), consider the following:

What practical help and information should Wendy be given at this time?

Wendy will need the support of a close relative or friend, and this person should be called into the department. A doctor should see Wendy to assess her state of shock, and possibly prescribe some form of sedation.

It will be necessary for a post-mortem to be performed on Charles Lewis to ascertain the exact cause of death and an inquest will probably be held some months later. There will be no immediate death certificate signed and no funeral can take place until the police give permission following the post-mortem. All Wendy can do at this stage, then, is to go home with her friend/relative and await a visit from the police. She may find support in the long term from associations such as Cruse (260 Sheen Road, Richmond, Surrey), formed with the aim of giving practical advice and emotional support to widows. Initially, however, information about such organizations is probably not appropriate and could almost certainly not be absorbed.

The police come to interview James Bryant, the driver of the car.

How do you feel about Mr Bryant?

It is true that Mr Bryant's actions have caused the death of a young man. It is also true that he may well be suffering the most tremendous personal guilt at the enormity of what has happened. It would be almost impossible to imagine the extent of his self-recrimination. He is also probably fairly frightened about the possible outcome of this incident for him. Mr Bryant's life, too, has been shattered at this point and laying blame would not be appropriate or constructive.

Had Wendy known for some time that her husband was going to die, and had she been able to prepare for the event, would her grief have followed a different pattern? (See Chaney 1980; Parkes 1980.)

The suddenness of Charles Lewis's death denied Wendy the chance of taking her leave of him as she may have wished. She may always regret her last words to him. Had Charles suffered an illness, and had they both been aware that Charles was going to die, then they could perhaps have grieved jointly and spent their final time together in a more positive manner.

Health carers, too, can take more satisfaction and feel more professional pride in caring for someone who they know is dying. There are fewer feelings of guilt when it is felt that relatives are given the support that they need.

Wendy is just as likely to experience the stages of grieving as any other widow. These stages may be timed differently (people who know that a relative is terminally ill tend to grieve before he/she dies) and Wendy may not experience all of the stages or may choose to suppress some of them.

This is true of people everywhere. Grief is a personal emotion and, whilst some aspects of grief have been identified and defined, each relative – and member of staff – will experience it in his or her own way.

DISCUSSION AND FURTHER STUDY

In this vignette we have really been addressing two issues. One is the matter of sudden death, the other is the matter of social drinking and driving.

We have not actually considered the problem of alcoholism. You will be able to find reference to this topic in the media and in current health care publications. (See, for instance, Minshull 1985, Mitchell 1985, Morris 1985.) The Alcohol Studies Centre, Paisley College of Technology, Westerfield Annexe, 25 High Calside, Paisley, PA2 6BY is also an informative resource.

As a point of further discussion, you may like to consider the following hypothesis.

The day following Charles Lewis's accident had been planned as the day for the Accident and Emergency Department's staff party. It takes place in the evening; many of the nursing and medical staff are drinking and are planning to drive home afterwards.

What ethical questions arise from this situation?

Discuss the personal and professional responsibilities of the member of staff at this party.

REFERENCES TO VIGNETTE 10

KEY REFERENCES

Chaney, P. S. (ed.) 1980. *Dealing with Death and Dying*. International Communications Inc., Pennsylvania.

Parkes, C. M. 1980. *Bereavement: Studies of Grief in Adult Life*. Pelican Books, London.

Wright, Bob. 1986. *Caring in Crisis*. Churchill Livingstone, Edinburgh.

ADDITIONAL REFERENCES

Minshull, D. 1985. Sick or self-indulgent? *Nursing Mirror*, 161(1), 3 July.

Mitchell, D. 1985. Defeating the demon. *Nursing Mirror*, 161(1), 3 July.

Morris, P. 1985. The dependent spirit. *Nursing Times*, Vol.81, pp.12–13, 6 February.

JONATHAN LONDON

Jonathan is a teenager who sniffs glue.

In this vignette and the next one we will be considering the concept of abuse.

What does this word mean to you?

With what other words do you most commonly associate it?

The many facets of abuse are today widely reported. It is not necessary to be working in the health care professions to have gained some insight into the phenomenon.

CHECK ▶ Before answering questions in the following vignette, it is necessary that you should understand the following:

1 ▶ The psychological aspects of adolescent development.

2 ▶ What is meant by the use of the term 'misuse of drugs'.

3 ▶ Some of the terms relating to the misuse of drugs, i.e. tolerance, withdrawal effects, dependance and addiction.

(See key references, page 156. Also the leaflets which have been produced by the Department of Health and Social Security. Relevant titles are 'Drug misuse, a basic briefing; 'What Parents can Do About Drugs' and 'Drugs: What You Can Do As a Parent'.)

Adolescence is a time for taking risks. It is a time for seeking peer group identity whilst establishing independence from the family. One way of emphasizing autonomy is to rebel against family and societal rules. Solvent abuse is an example of such a rebellion.

Ellen Murray is a school nurse who has come to test 14-year-old children to see if it would be advisable for them to be vaccinated against TB. She also uses this as an opportunity to try to detect any obvious health problems. She meets Jonathan London who gives her some cause for concern. He appears very thin, lacks concentration and his eyes are slightly blood-shot. He also seems very hostile.

Admittedly, Ellen may not usually have picked this up after one short meeting, but teachers were concerned at the change of behaviour in this intelligent, normally alert boy, and had asked Ellen to look out for him.

Ellen writes to Jonathan's mother and asks her to accompany him when he comes back for the administration of the BCG vaccination, should it prove necessary. At this meeting Ellen asks Mrs London whether she has noticed any change in Jonathan's moods. Mrs London says, 'Well, yes, but it is his age and only to be expected.' Ellen explains that the teachers have been very concerned about Jonathan. She also says that while examining him in her capacity as school nurse she suspected he might be taking drugs or glue sniffing. Mrs London is absolutely horrified and utterly denies that this could be possible.

When challenged, Jonathan is adamant that he has never taken drugs. When pressed, it is with some relief that he admits to what he sees as the lesser charge of solvent abuse.

Mrs London is initially very cross with him and cannot understand why her son should have chosen to demonstrate this behaviour. Ellen decides to make time to discuss this matter at some length with Mrs London, and she makes an appointment to see her the next morning at the Health Centre.

How would you answer Mrs London's very obvious questions of Why? How? What should I be looking out for?

(Gay, M. 1986 will help you to formulate these answers.)

Only Jonathan can actually tell his mother why he started glue-sniffing. It may help Mrs London to realize that she is not alone in her problem, and that at this stage it is something which is relatively easy to control. She is likely to be feeling very guilty, and there really is little you can say to help her in this respect.

Many youngsters probably start glue-sniffing from curiosity, or because their friends are doing it. Others like taking risks, particularly if they know their parents, or other adults, would disapprove. It may be that Jonathan is bored. He may be depressed, worried or resentful about family or school problems. He may have been glue-sniffing as a cry of help to attract attention. Certainly, the fact that Jonathan has admitted fairly readily that he is abusing solvents is a hopeful sign. It would seem that he is ready to be helped.

We have discussed some of Jonathan's symptoms. In conversation Ellen manages to get a fuller picture about Jonathan's change of moods. What sort of problems do you think Mrs London may mention at this point?

(Watson, J. 1987 is particularly informative.)

Jonathan has displayed a loss of appetite and he has been very tired and exhausted. Mrs London has been aware from his school reports that his work has deteriorated and there have been a couple of occasions when she realized that he had not been to school at all. Jonathan had been coming in late at night and on one occasion he even stayed out all night. Mrs London says that, having thought about it overnight, she has been aware that seemingly unrelated, unimportant articles have been missing from the house. She had put it down to her own forgetfulness rather than the fact that somebody may have been taking them. The articles she described are those typically used by young solvent abusers, e.g. shoe polish, hair spray, nail polish remover, glue, freezer bags and binliners. On one or two occasions Mrs London says she has lost small amounts of money and did at one point wonder whether perhaps Jonathan had 'borrowed them'.

Ellen asks Mrs London how far she thinks the problem has gone. Mrs London says she couldn't actually say, and this is something that Jonathan would have to answer. On a couple of evenings, however, when Jonathan came home late his speech was very slurred and he seemed somewhat aggressive. Mr and Mrs London had thought that their son was drunk. Although they were not pleased about it they decided it was just a natural part of growing up.

What satisfaction do you think young people get from the abuse of solvents?

The experience is very much like being drunk; youngsters get together and fool about. Dreamlike experiences may occur; generally these are not true hallucinations as youngsters don't confuse them with reality. The effects of solvent vapours come on quickly and disappear within a few minutes to half an hour after the sniffing has stopped. Afterwards the youngster may experience a mild hangover for about a day.

Ellen decides to speak to Jonathan about his problem, and Mrs London is very happy for this to happen. Ellen asks Jonathan exactly how he goes about inhaling solvents, how frequently he does it, and whether he does it on his own. At the last question Jonathan seems very defensive. It's obvious that he does not want to be seen to be getting any of his friends into trouble. He says that he usually sniffs glue by putting it into an empty crisp bag, placing this over his mouth and nose and inhaling it.

From your reading, have you learned about any other methods of inhaling solvents?

The practice of saturating a rag or sweatband with solvents such as turpentine or antifreeze is fairly common. Some youngsters practise the very dangerous habit of placing a polythene bag over their heads and holding the solvent inside. This method is usually used by those who prefer aerosols such as hair lacquer.

What do you think Ellen should now do about Jonathan? How can she most effectively help him?

Ellen could refer Jonathan to a dependency unit attached to the local hospital if there is one. You may like to find out what facilities there are in your area. She could proceed and support the London family herself if this is what they wish.

Probably the most useful approach to take is one of counselling about how to plan gradual weaning away from dependency without demanding immediate abstinence and without threats of punishment. It is really a case of Jonathan organizing his life and looking for other things to do when he would otherwise have been sniffing glue. If, for example, he was formally an active partaker in sport, it may be that he would like to take this up again.

The very long-term, heavy solvent misuser may develop moderate, lasting impairment of brain function affecting especially the control of movement. Chronic misuse of aerosols and cleaning fluid has caused lasting kidney and liver damage, while repeatedly sniffing lead in petrol may result in lead poisoning. It may be worth warning Jonathan of these long-term effects, although if he is not feeling in a receptive mood it may have no effect on him whatsoever.

Possibly the most important, and yet the most difficult, aim will be to help Mr and Mrs London during this time. If they constantly nag Jonathan, it may reinforce his feeling that he wants to alienate himself from his parents, and this will not help at all. It is probably more important that they monitor their son's health, to see whether the worrying signs occur less or more frequently.

Prevention is better than cure. What strategies for the prevention of solvent abuse have you become aware of?

Do you think that high profiling the situation on television, for example, is effective or does it in fact exacerbate the situation?

This is a tremendous social problem. Glue and other solvents are easily obtainable, even though most shops now clearly display notices saying that they ban the sale of solvents to children under the age of eighteen.

External agencies such as the police, representatives of the health service and the social work department can be of considerable assistance to schools teaching such programmes, since they can provide practical and realistic views of the problem.

FURTHER STUDENT ACTIVITY

As a small project, you may like to look at the national picture of drug abuse which is current as you read this book.

It could be said that the Londons are lucky that Jonathan has not become a drug abuser. There is much written about this problem, and the reference leaflets will be of great help to you here.

Can you identify what these drug-related slang terms mean?

Speed	Magic mushrooms
Pot	Dikes
Dope	One, One Eights
Hash	Acid
Grass	Tranquillisers
Coke	Injecting
Smack	
Skag	

The DHSS leaflets outlined on page 152 will explain these words.

---

1   Are you aware of any health education programmes in your district, warning people about the hazards of drug taking?
2   What facilities are there available in your area to support drug abusers?

REFERENCES TO VIGNETTE 11

KEY REFERENCES

Cameron, J. 1987. Hidden dangers. *Nursing Times*, 18 March, pp.59–60.

Gay, M. 1986. Drug and solvent abuse in adolescence. *Nursing Times*, 19 January, pp.34–5.

Morton et al. 1983. Solvent abuse. *Nursing Mirror, Community Forum 10*, 14 December, pp.i–iv.

Ron, M. 1986. Volatile substance abuse. *British Journal of Psychiatry*, vol.148, pp.235–46.

Stuart, P. 1986. Solvents and schoolchildren. *Health Education Journal*, Vol.45(2), pp.84–6.

Watson, J. 1987. *Solvent Abuse. The adolescent epidemic?* Croom Helm, Kent.

JANETTE AND BARRY MARTINS

Janette finds the strain of caring for two small children overwhelming.

We have briefly discussed one aspect of abuse – abuse of self. In recent years, public awareness concerning the abuse of children has been heightened.

What are your personal feelings about people who abuse their children? You may like to discuss this with your colleagues.

CHECK ▶

Before answering the questions in the following vignette you should explore and discuss the following:

1 ▶ Normal child development.

2 ▶ What is meant by the 'at risk' register.

3 ▶ Current media reports relating to the abuse of children.
(You will find that reading newspapers and magazines will probably provide you with much information about the current situation relating to child abuse. See also key references, page 160.)

Janette and Barry Martins have two children, one aged 2½ years and one aged 3 months.

Using your knowledge of child development, describe the children's predicted physical activities at these ages.
(A useful reference here is Sheriden 1975.)

Barry is a business executive whose work occasionally takes him from home. Belinda, the 2½-year-old toddler, is very active. She will be starting play-group as soon as she is three but at the moment there is no vacancy for her. She is full of mischief, rarely rests and Janette often feels that she cannot predict what Belinda will do next. By the time she goes to bed at night, Janette is exhausted.

Oliver, the baby, has not yet developed the pattern of sleeping through the night. Janette gets frustrated because he will wake for a feed (Janette is breast feeding), settle down, but then start to cry about half an hour later for no apparent reason.

One night, when Barry is away, it all gets too much for Janette. She picks Oliver up shakes him hard and in her frustration throws him against the cot side. The pattern is repeated the following night, only this time Janette throws Oliver down the stairs. When Barry gets home the following evening he cannot help but notice the bruises on his son's arms, a slight bruise on his face and some darker bruising on his body. He asks Janette what happened and she says, 'I fell down the stairs while I was carrying him.'

Barry is very concerned and decides to take the child to the local Accident and Emergency Department for a check-up.

What are your feelings about Janette's behaviour at this point?

In the Accident and Emergency Department, Oliver is given a thorough check-up, but there appear to be no fractures and he has apparently sustained no head injury. However, there is concern on the part of the staff nurse who is caring for Oliver as she suspects possible child abuse.

What are the signs of child abuse? (A useful reference here is Smith 1976.)

Possible signs are:

1 Unexplained cuts and bruises. It is important to remember that toddlers often get these, but babies do not. The alert health carer will be on the look-out for unlikely explanations.
2 Repeated minor injuries are a possible indication of abuse.
3 Scalds and burns, particularly cigarette burns, are suspect.
4 Fractures, lacerations and swellings.
5 Human bites.
6 Facial bruising, loose teeth, swollen lips.
7 Failure to thrive, weight loss, withdrawal or aggression, slow development, tiredness and lethargy.
8 Unexplained abscesses.
9 Excessive crying.
10 Attitude of parents, either unfeeling or perhaps over-anxious.

Staff nurse's suspicions may also have been aroused because there has been some delay between the reported time of the injury and the time of attendance at the Accident and Emergency Department. This is Oliver's first attendance here; had he attended frequently before then staff nurse's suspicions would have been even more acute. Nevertheless she is concerned because there does not seem to be an adequate or a likely explanation for Oliver's injuries.

Look at your district policy on child abuse. What may now be the procedure?

As long as the medical and nursing staff have any suspicions that this child has been abused, it is likely that he will be admitted to hospital. Barry is told that Oliver is to be admitted for observation overnight. He does not refuse this, but had he done so it is possible that the paediatrician and social worker would have been contacted. If it's deemed to be necessary, a child may be admitted into hospital under a safety order. If necessary the police may be contacted.

A child who is thought to have been abused may be entered into the child abuse register. This is most commonly maintained by the local NSPCC special unit on behalf of an area review committee. Its purposes are as follows:

1   To provide detailed readily available information about children known or suspected to have suffered abuse.
2   To aid the diagnosis of a sequence of repeated injuries which might otherwise have been unrelated and not seen as repeated abuse.
3   To avoid unnecessary duplication of a service to the child and family and aid good communication between the two agencies.
4   To provide a basis for regular monitoring of the child and family.
5   To provide statistical data on the incidence of child abuse for planning purposes and to provide material for training and research.

There are set criteria for the inclusion for children under 17 on the At Risk Register. Perhaps you could find out what the criteria are for your district. *The local NSPCC may help you here, or indeed the information may be available in your own Accident and Emergency Department.*

A child is included or removed from the register at a case conference. Staff who may be involved in the Area Review Committee to whom the At Risk Register is always available are hospital doctors, GPs, social workers, the NSPCC, police, nurseries and play-groups, head teachers and education welfare offciers, community nursing staff and probation officers. Representatives of these agencies will also be present at case conferences.

Do you think Oliver's name should be entered on the At Risk Register?

You may like to discuss this with your colleagues and it would be relevant to refer to PAIN, a pressure group set up by Steve and Sue Amphlett. PAIN stands for Parents Against Injustice, as Steve's and Sue's young daughter had a spate of accidents and ended up on the child abuse register. The social worker called and even discussed taking the children into care!

It was found that the Amphletts' daughter had brittle bones.

Oliver's name is placed on the At Risk Register for a few months until he is one year old. Barry Martin is so horrified that he looks at ways of supporting his wife and does not leave her alone with the children when he has to go away on business.

This story has a happy ending in that the At Risk Register served its purpose. It prevented Oliver coming to any more harm and Janette was helped to get through a very difficult period.

FURTHER DISCUSSION AND SUMMARY

Having briefly considered the needs of one family where frustration rather than habitual abuse has led to measures being taken on the part of the State, you may like to consider the following.

1 What do you see as being the rights of the child, the rights of the parent, and the rights of the State in such a situation?
2 Contact the NSPCC. See if you can find out what their action is in the case of suspected child abuse.
3 Read the following articles if you can obtain them:
   (a) 'The legacy of Maria Colwell,' *Social Work Today*, vol. 10, No. 19.
   (b) 'Death of a child,' *New Society*, vol. 39, No. 752.
4 Perhaps you would now like to consider child sexual abuse. Much is currently being written about this and the activities of the pressure groups such as 'Childline' was widely publicized. A useful article as an introduction to this topic is published in the *Nursing Times/Mirror*, 15 January 1986, p. 16.

REFERENCES TO VIGNETTE 12

KEY REFERENCES

Bedford, A. 1985. Child abuse: the A & E nurses' role. *Nursing Mirror*, 23 October, pp.20–22.

Brooks, L. 1985. A vicious circle. *Nursing Times*, 10 July, pp.32–5

Dingwall, R. 1983a. Detecting child abuse. *Nursing Times*, 15 June, pp.26–30.

Dingwall, R. 1983b. Child abuse. *Nursing Times*, 22 June, pp.67–8.

Edwards, K. 1987. Probing the power struggle. *Nursing Times*, 83(17), 29 April, pp.47–51.

Evans, R. 1985. The silent victims. *Nursing Times*, 27 November, pp.59–60.

McAree, J. 1987. A family affair. *Nursing Times*, 2 April, pp.66–9.

Powall, M. A. 1985. A family affair? *Nursing Times*, 23 October, pp.58–61.

Sadler, C. 1986. The forgotten children. *Nursing Times*, 26 November, pp.16–17.

Walsh, M. 1986. Counting the bruises. *Nursing Times*, 17 September, pp.62–4.

ADDITIONAL REFERENCES

Sheriden, M. 1975. *From Birth to Five Years*. N.F.E.R., Nelson, London.

Smith, S. 1976. *The Battered Child Syndrome*. Butterworth, London.

IAN METCALFE

Ian fractures a femur and is in hospital for three months.

In this chapter we will be considering the needs of Ian, a 17-year-old who is suddenly admitted to hospital and whose condition necessitates a lengthy period of confinement to bed.

Have you ever nursed anyone in a similar situation? How did he or she react?

CHECK ▶ Before proceeding with this narrative, make sure that you have investigated and understand the following:

1 ▶ The structure, position and function of the femur.

2 ▶ The way in which broken bones heal.

3 ▶ The process of passing from childhood to adulthood. (See key references, page 167 for suggested reading.)

Ian Metalfe has sustained a fractured shaft of the right femur in a road traffic accident. This is being treated by skeletal traction and it is anticipated that Ian will be in hospital for about twelve weeks.

Before going any further, stop and make sure that you have an understanding of what skeletal traction is. The relevant key references will help you, particularly the Nursing Times Service publication. (1973).

Ian has been a patient on the orthopaedic ward for three days.

With reference to your reading, and remembering Ian's age and the unexpected predicament in which he finds himself, what do you think his concerns may be at this time?

His concerns may be related to the nature of his illness, pain which he may be experiencing, fears for his future mobility.

You may have considered that at his age a lack of privacy and exposure may worry and indeed embarrass him. His admission to hospital at such a time could interfere with his struggle for independence from his family. Alternatively, separation from the security of peers, family and school may make him feel very insecure. Ian will almost certainly be feeling threatened by an overwhelming sense of helplessness.

Anxiety or embarrassment at the loss of control could be expressed by anger, depression or insecurity. He may actually reject treatment or procedures. The antithesis of this may be that he becomes very dependent on the staff and appears to be very dependent on his parents who visit him. During the initial period of his admission he may appear very withdrawn in an attempt to deny to himself that he actually is in this unenviable situation.

Ian's accident occurred when he crashed a newly purchased motor cycle which he persuaded his parents to buy for him following many protracted arguments. His motor cycle was 'written off' during the accident, and Ian spends much of his time bemoaning the fate of his beloved vehicle.

Why do you think the motor cycle was so important to Ian at this age?

Ian's motor cycle had probably provided him with a very necessary means of transport, and possibly gave him independence from his parents and friends. If you have any understanding of adolescent development, you may have identified the fact that this is the time for the development of a self-concept. There is a search for an identity and a role. If Ian's motor cycle had formed a part of the role which he had designed for himself, then to lose it could equally destroy his developing self-image.

Having built up a picture of Ian and his needs, imagine you are on the ward caring for him and consider the following:

What nursing intervention do you consider would be appropriate to prevent Ian developing physical problems, bearing in mind that he is in a position which will prevent any movement of his right leg for about twelve weeks, that the end of his bed will be elevated so that he is lying at an angle, and that a metal pin will have been driven through his bone to provide a point of attachment for the traction apparatus?

Ian will almost certainly experience some pain in the first few days following his accident. This pain will be related primarily to the muscles surrounding the fracture as these will be contracting at this time. The medical staff will almost definitely have prescribed analgesia and muscle relaxants, and the nursing intervention should be planned to administer these with view to preventing pain before it occurs.

Because of the angle at which he has to lie, Ian may well have problems of elimination. Urine tends to stagnate in the bladder, causing urinary retention and consequent urinary tract infection; inadequacies of diet, coupled with the difficulty of using bed pans in this position, may lead to constipation. A high fibre diet, rich in vitamin C to promote bone healing, is the ideal.

Ian is obviously prone to becoming very sore and it is particularly his shoulders, skin around any splint which may have been applied, and his left heel, which he will probably be using as a lever, which need special attention.

Nursing intervention must also clearly be aimed at helping Ian to keep himself clean. He will probably be able to wash his own face and hands and indeed the front half of his upper trunk, but will certainly need help with washing his back, his buttocks, his left leg and as much of his right leg as possible. Anyone confined to bed will probably find it very comforting to be able to soak his own hands and feet in a bowl of water whenever this can be arranged. It is likely that Ian will be able to attend to cleaning his own teeth, but he may well need help with washing his hair.

Next time you are working on a ward where there are male patients, look to see how many mirrors are provided for the men so that they may shave and do their own hair as they would wish to.

The situation could arise where a patient's standards of hygiene do not meet your own. Supposing, for example, that Ian does not wish to clean his teeth and says he only does it once or twice a week at home.

You may wish to discuss this situation with your colleagues. Do you think you have any right to expect Ian to conform to your personal standards of hygiene? Do you have any responsibilities as a nurse to educate him about dental hygiene?

There is a general agreement among the ward staff that Ian is rather bad tempered and aggressive.

Can you suggest any reasons for this? (Spielberger 1979 is a particularly relevant reference here.)

One morning when you are assisting Ian with his daily wash, he offends you with his use of sexually explicit language and with the 'personal' suggestions he makes to you. Can you imagine how you would feel in this situation, and how you would deal with it?

Ian's offensive language and unwelcome advances may remind you of situations with which you are personally familiar. There is no 'right' response to the question posed but in order to clarify your thinking it may help you to refer back to the ethical decision-making model given in chapter six. This should help you to list and consider the alternative actions which could be taken, together with their probable outcomes. Do remember, though, that one of the purposes of thought clarification is to lessen your personal guilts and to remind you that, as an individual, you have rights.

Two phone calls are made to the ward concerning Ian. One is from the local newspaper. A journalist is enquiring about the accident, how it occurred, and Ian's present condition. Another phone call is from the local police station; a policeman wishes to visit Ian to take a statement.

What would the correct response be in each of these situations?
Check the policy in the district where you are now working.

A third phone call is received from Ian's mother, who is naturally very anxious and wishes to visit her son whom she hasn't seen since the previous day. Part of Ian's aggression is focused upon his parents and he has said many times during the day that if his parents wish to visit he does not wish to see them.

Bearing in mind Ian's age, does he have the right to refuse to see his parents?

Do nurses have the right to influence his decision?

If you have found that you are unsure about the issue of confidentiality and of patients' and relatives' rights then refer back to the chapter in this book which looks at legal issues in nursing.

Young, A. P. 1981. *Legal Problems in Nursing Practice.* Harper and Row will also provide the information which you require.

Ian's general reluctance to comply with his treatment is again noted when he refuses to exercise his limbs and shows a marked unwillingness to change his position in bed.

Why are exercise and movement important for Ian's recovery, and how can he be helped to understand this?

Movement is clearly an essential component in the prevention of pressure sores. Movement of uninjured limbs is crucial. When Ian does eventually get out of bed he will need strong arms in order to use crutches, and a very strong left leg which will have to support him for as long as his right leg is non-weight bearing. If these limbs are not exercised during the period in which Ian is confined to bed, muscle wasting will occur and his limbs will be of very little use to him.

If you have worked on an orthopaedic ward, make a list of all the staff who were involved in the patient's recovery. If you have not worked on an orthopaedic ward yet, perhaps you would like to identify some people who you think may be involved in Ian's recovery.

Apart from the doctors and nurses, physiotherapists, occupational therapists, radiographers and social workers play a vital role in the recovery of patients on an orthopaedic ward. The main aim of caring for a person in hospital is to restore him to health and to get him home as soon as possible. Ian's rehabilitation programme should begin very early during his hospitalization.

What role do you think each of the health caring professions would play in Ian's recovery? If you are not sure of the answer perhaps you would like to discuss this with the non-nursing and non-medical staff that you meet both within the hospital and the community.

DISCUSSION AND FURTHER STUDY

We have considered some of the problems of a young man who has suddenly been admitted to hospital, and the impact this has upon him.

His moods may, of course, be related to his age, although pain, fear, embarrassment, boredom and unhappiness will also be contributing factors. These latter factors may be particularly important if there are no other patients of Ian's age in the ward.

It is worth remembering, too, that patients of Ian's age may well still be students who are studying for A level or other examinations or indeed they may have recently commenced new jobs. In days of unemployment, a prolonged period of absence from a new job may seem, and indeed may be, disastrous.

STUDENT ACTIVITY

1   You may like to discuss and share with your colleagues your opinions about mixed sex wards. Are they desirable? Should patients of similar ages be nursed together or are 'family' groupings more suitable? Do resources within the health service enable there to be any choice for patients or staff in this matter?

2   Check that you understand the purpose of skeletal traction. What other types of traction are there? When would skin traction be applied in preference to skeletal traction?

3   Look at the diagram opposite. This shows one form of Skeletal traction. What is the function of the ropes labelled A, B, C in this diagram? (The referenced text by Crawford Adams 1978 will help you to answer this problem.)

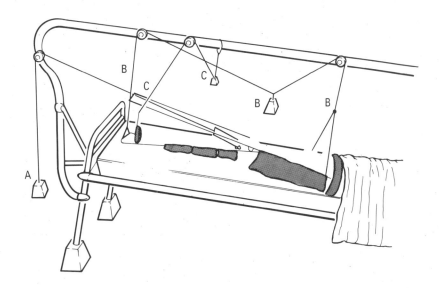

4 Use Roper's (1985) model of nursing as a framework to identify Ian's needs.

5 Refer back to the chapter on nursing management in which some models of nursing are outlined. Orem's self-help model may well be an appropriate framework for planning Ian's care. Perhaps you would like to plan Ian's care for the third day of his stay in hospital.

REFERENCES TO VIGNETTE 13

KEY REFERENCES

A) ON ADOLESCENCE

Conger, J. 1979. *Adolescence: A Generation under Pressure.* Harper & Row, London.

Henrikson, B. 1983. *Not for Sale:* Young People in Society. Aberdeen University Press, Scotland.

Law, C. 1985. An anguished adolescent. *Nursing Times,* 9 January, pp.40–43.

Law, C. 1985 Physiological changes in adolescence. *Nursing: The Add-On Journal of Clinical Nursing,* 2(40), August, pp.1173, 1175–7.

Lowe, G. R. 1979. *The Growth of Personality: Infancy to Old Age.* Penguin Books, London.

Mayle, P. 1982. *'What's Happening to Me'?* Macmillan, London.

Sanwick, M. 1985. Psychological adjustment in adolescence. *Nursing: The Add-on Journal of Clinical Nursing*, 2(40), August, pp.1179–81.

Open University. 1982. *Parents and Teenagers*. Harper & Row, London.

B) ON FRACTURES

Crawford-Adams, J. 1978a. *An Outline of Fractures*. Churchill Livingstone, Edinburgh.

Crawford-Adams, J. 1978b. *An Outline of Orthopaedics*. Churchill-Livingstone, Edingburgh.

Nursing Times Service. 1973. *Understanding Traction*. Macmillan, London.

Pinney, E. 1983. *Orthopaedic Nursing*. Baillière Tindall, London.

C) ON STRESS

Bailey, R. D. 1985. *Coping with Stress*. Blackwell, Oxford.

Burrows, R. 1984. Nurses and violence. *Nursing Times*, 25 January, Vol. 80, pp.56–8.

Moran, J. 1984. Aggression management . *Nursing Times*, 4 April, Vol. 80, pp.28–31.

Spielberger, C. 1979. *Psychological Reaction to Illness and Health*. Harper & Row, New York.

Wilson-Barnett, J. 1979. *Stress In Hospital*. Churchill Livingstone, Edinburgh.

**ADDITIONAL
REFERENCES**

For guidance for models on nursing, see:
Aggleton, P. and Chalmers, H. 1985. Models and theories. Orem's self-care model. *Nursing Times*, 81(1), pp.36–9.

Chapman, C. M. 1985. *Theory of Nursing*. Lippincott Series, Harper & Row, London.

Miller, A. 1985. Theories in nursing. *Nursing Times*, 8(10), p.14.

Pearson, A., and Vaughan, B. 1980. *Nursing Models for Practice*. Heinemann, London.

SYLVIA NORMAN

Sylvia is experiencing an acute episode of cystitis.

In this section, we will be considering the role of the nurse as a health educator in the community by focusing on the needs of a woman who is suffering from cystitis.

Have you ever suffered from cystitis yourself?

Do you know of anyone who has?

What symptoms do you associate with cystitis?

How do you feel when non-nursing friends ask you for advice relating to health problems?

These are all questions which you may like to ask yourself, or discuss with colleagues, before continuing the study.

The last question particularly may benefit from peer group discussion.

Possible reactions to this could be:

'I feel threatened or embarrassed because I may not know the answer.'
'I feel flattered.'
'I feel worried and/or responsible in case I give bad advice.'
'I feel cross to have been asked when I'm off duty.'

Any of these responses could be appropriate and indeed being asked to give advice can put one in an invidious situation. The only 'golden rule', probably, is that if you're unsure then don't give any advice at all, but refer your friend to someone who knows.

CHECK ▶ Before attempting to answer the questions posed, you should make sure that you understand and investigate the following:

1 ▶ The structure of the female urinary tract;

2 ▶ The constituents of urine;

3 ▶ The meaning of the term cystitis. (See Kilmartin 1973, 1980, and other sources cited in the key references on page 176.)

Late one night, Sylvia Norman, a young woman living in the flat below you, hammers on your door, wakes you up and says that she is in agony but does not like to disturb her GP! She says she feels sure that this is cystitis as she had a similar, although less painful, attack some years ago.

What symptoms have you, from your reading, learned to associate with cystitis?

Your neighbour describes her symptoms in these terms: 'I have to keep getting up to pass water and it's agony. Last time, I thought I wouldn't make it to the toilet soon enough, but there was nothing to pass when I got there. When I do pass water it's very thick which is what happened when I had cystitis before.' You notice that she looks flushed, and when you ask her about the pain, she says that it's her 'tummy' which hurts most although her back is now starting to ache as well.

Kilmartin, in both her books, points out that cystitis is very difficult to define, and that the term is sometimes used as an umbrella term for all bladder problems and infections.

True cystitis, as defined by Kilmartin, has three symptoms:

1 pain when passing urine;
2 frequency when passing urine;
3 sometimes blood loss when passing urine.

It is important to distinguish bladder infection, which produces the above symptoms, from infection of the urethra, or urethritis.

'First-aid' at the commencement of these symptoms will prevent the development of urethritis, in which the pain on passing urine becomes so great that it is totally unbearable and can even send the sufferer into a state of clinical shock. The passing of blood indicates the infection has spread from the bladder to the urethra.

Using your knowledge of anatomy and physiology, consider the following:

If untreated, where else could the infection spread to, and what would the possible consequences be? Watson and Royle (1987) will help you here.

From the bladder, the infection could progress up the ureters to the kidneys, bringing a dull ache, a temperature and general malaise. Any scarring in the kidneys caused by bacteria may cause permanent reduction of kidney function – albeit minute!

What, in relation to Sylvia, are your short- and long-term goals for helping her? Try to work this out for yourself, although either of Kilmartin's books has the relevant information.

The first aim must be for the immediate 'first aid' treatment, which aims to 'flush out' any infection, thus reducing infection and pain.

There is much you can do to relieve an attack of cystitis. Of course, your neighbour has had it before and may have found her own way of relieving the pain and discomfort of an attack, so you could ask her about this. It is usually easier to make people comfortable in their own surroundings, so you may suggest to her that you go to her flat. You could then instigate the following regime which she will, in fact, probably be able to manage herself.

1   **Attack** the infection by asking your neighbour to drink a pint of water immediately. Warn her that this drink is the first of many and that, although water is best, she may prefer to drink squash, milk or weak tea. Tell her that she needs to keep a supply of liquid at hand.

2   **Relieve** the pain.
(a)   Hot water bottles can be very comforting and relieve pain locally. If possible get two ready, so that your neighbour can put one on her lower back and the other between her thighs. (Remember to wrap the bottles in towels so that the skin is not burned.)
(b)   Mix a teaspoon of bicarbonate of soda with some water for your neighbour to drink. Suggest that she repeats this every hour for the next three hours.

What effects will sodium bicarbonate have?

Should you have any reservations about advising anyone to take it?

Sodium bicarbonate reduces the acidity of the urine, and so relieves some of the burning pain on urination. The bacteria causing the infection which precipitates cystitis will stop multiplying. Bicarbonate of soda does not taste particularly nice, and your neighbour may need some persuasion to drink the solution. (*A cautionary note*: anyone suffering from hypertension would be ill advised to take sodium bicarbonate, so you should ensure that your neighbour does not have this problem.)
(c)   Two mild analgesic tablets, if your neighbour has some which she normally takes, may help.

3   **Attack** the infection again. As soon as she can manage it, your neighbour should drink another half to one pint of water. Advise her to repeat this every twenty minutes.

She may be reluctant to do this as it will cause her to pass urine frequently and urination will be painful. However, you can honestly say that the pain usually lessens as time passes and it is essential to keep emptying the bladder in order to 'flush out' the harmful bacteria.

4   **Rest and relaxation** Suggest to your neighbour that she should make herself as comfortable as possible with the hot water bottles in a bed or an armchair as near to the toilet as possible. A jug of water should be kept close to hand, as your neighbour should keeping drinking

about ½ pint every twenty minutes for at least three hours. Three hours is a long time to endure the pain and discomfort of cystitis, so if you don't feel that you can stay to keep your neighbour company, suggest that she keeps herself occupied with a book or a crossword. If she follows the regime which has been described, your neighbour's cystitis should subside within three hours.

Your 'first aid' treatment is effective and the next day your neighbour tells you that she feels fully recovered and that she knows what to do next time she has 'an attack'. This would be a useful opportunity to explain how cystitis occurs and how she may be able to prevent further 'attacks'. Your neighbour gratefully accepts your offer to discuss this with her.

As an exercise, describe the female urinary system to nursing colleagues. How many words do you use which may not make sense to anyone who has minimal or no understanding of anatomy?

Your neighbour may not, for example, understand the word bladder, and you may find yourself talking in terms of the 'bag which holds the urine'. You might even have to explain what urine is! You may well find yourself talking in terms of 'back passages' and 'front passages'. Avoid being patronizing though; Sylvia may be fully conversant with all the anatomical terms which you need to use. Diagrams sometimes help, if you can draw, but a poor diagram will only confuse.

Using the referenced texts plan a discussion which you could have with your neighbour in which you address the following questions:

What is cystitis?
What causes it?
What may prevent it?

One way of expressing this information in everyday terms could be as follows.

WHAT IS CYSTITIS?

Cystitis is an inflammation inside the bladder. Over half the women in this country suffer from it at some time during their lives, often repeatedly.

WHAT CAUSES IT?

There are several things which can cause an inflammation of the bladder including germs, allergic reactions and friction.

GERMS (BACTERIA)

Cystitis can be caused by germs which normally live in and around the bowel opening. Sometimes they get into the water passage and bladder, which are normally germ free. Once inside the bladder the germs multiply and irritate its lining, causing inflammation.

In a woman the entrances to the water passage, vagina and anus are all very close so germs can travel very easily. This is why more women suffer from cystitis than men. The germs can be pushed into the water passage and bladder by sexual intercourse, by inserting tampons, by wiping your bottom from back to front, or even by wearing tight trousers. Common vaginal infections like thrush can also cause an attack of cystitis symptoms. And the germs which cause sexually transmitted diseases like herpes or trichomonas are sometimes responsible.

ALLERGIES

Some people find they are allergic to toiletries like vaginal deodorants, perfumed soap or talcum powder.

FRICTION OF THE WATER PASSAGE

The water passage is close to the vagina so this can happen during sexual intercourse.

Also, 'irritable bladder' a particularly sensitive bladder, or anxiety or depression can trigger off cystitis.

HOW TO PREVENT FURTHER ATTACKS

Drink at least three to four pints of liquids every day. This may seem a lot but it will help flush out any germs before they can get a grip.

Pass water whenever you feel the need. Try not to hang on – this can encourage an attack of cystitis. Count to twenty after passing water then strain again to push out the last drops.

If you find you get cystitis after sexual intercourse, try washing before and after intercourse and get your partner to do the same. (Of course, if you know your neighbour well, it may be easier to talk about sexual intercourse in terms of 'when John stays for the night'.) It might also help to pass water before and after. Some people find it helps to use a lubricant to prevent soreness and bruising. You can get this from chemists without prescription.

Always wipe your bottom from front to back. This helps stop germs spreading from the anus. Keep the genital area clean by washing yourself morning and night.

Don't use antiseptics, talcum powder, perfumed soap or deodorants in the genital area. Instead of perfumed soap, try unperfumed. And don't use shampoo or bath oils in the bath if you find they irritate.

If you get cystitis after drinking coffee, tea or alcohol, try diluting them or avoid them altogether.

Avoid wearing tight trousers. And try to wear cotton pants and tights with a cotton gusset. Man-made fibres don't allow your skin to breathe so easily and may irritate. You may prefer to wear stockings rather than tights.

What would you say to your neighbour if she asks you if or when she should consult her GP?

It's impossible to give strict guidelines on how long Sylvia should wait before she goes to her doctor. She will probably be able to tell whether self-treatment is clearing up her cystitis or not. But in general, she should always see a doctor:

(a)   If an attack of cystitis continues for longer than a day or two despite self-treatment, or if she has repeated attacks. This is because it is possible for the infection to spread to the kidneys.
(b)   If she is pregnant. Pregnant women are particularly at risk of kidney infection.
(c)   If she notices blood in her urine.

NB: An attack of cystitis in men and children is uncommon and should always be referred to a doctor.

WHAT THE DOCTOR CAN DO

The doctor will probably ask for a urine sample to find out whether the cystitis is caused by germs. If it is, he will prescribe a course of antibiotics or other drugs depending on whether it is a bacterial or non-bacterial infection. If not, Sylvia may only need further advice on self-treatment and prevention.

If Sylvia also has a vaginal discharge or itch, her doctor may take a swab from her vagina to find out whether there are any germs there which need treatment.

If the cystitis doesn't clear up after treatment from her own doctor, Sylvia may be referred to a hospital. This is usually only necessary after repeated and persistent attacks of cystitis.

You may think of other questions which your neighbour may ask. I can only think of one more, and that is what she should do if she suspects that her cystitis is caused by a sexually transmitted disease.

How would you answer this question?

A suitable reply would be as follows.

If you think your cystitis could be caused by a sexually transmitted disease you can go direct to a genito-urinary medicine clinic (also known as a 'special' or VD clinic), especially if you have recently changed sexual partners or if a sexual partner complains of similar symptoms to yours. It is often possible to telephone the clinic in advance to make an appointment. You can find the number in the telephone directory under venereal diseases.

If you are given a course of drugs by your own doctor or at the clinic, it's a good idea to check whether your partner should be treated as well. Your partner will not necesarily have any symptoms but might have an infection which is causing your cystitis.

DISCUSSION AND FURTHER STUDY

We have considered the needs of a lady whose cystitis is relatively mild. Reading either of Kilmartin's books will have convinced you, I'm sure, of the way in which this condition, which the Health Education Authority claims effects over half Britain's women, can ruin a life and precipitate severe depression.

> 'Worsening means increasing pain in the urethra, frequent visits to the toilet to the point where you daren't get up from the seat, and even smears of blood on the toilet paper . . . The pain is not simply 'burning' glass but is like a minor operation without an anaesthetic . . . What is worse you cannot bathe it or soothe it like an external cut'. (Angela Kilmartin 1973)

You should be aware, too, that cystitis can affect children although the cause is usually allergy or hygiene related.

STUDENT ACTIVITY

1 Can you think of any occasions on which friends have asked you for health advice?
How did you respond?
Is there any way in which you feel you could have answered more effectively?
What do you think was good about your response?

2 With your colleagues, discuss the role of the nurse as an effective health educator even when she is off duty. For example, do you think nurses should smoke, thus endorsing the notion that this is a healthy thing to do?

3 Reconsider the structured, specific step-by-step advice which has been given to Sylvia. Think of another area where friends or neighbours may ask you for advice and, using the same approach, plan what you would say.

REFERENCES TO VIGNETTE 14

KEY REFERENCES

Fisk, Dr P. 1982. *Pocket Guide to Cystitis*. Arlington Books, London.

Health Education Council. *Cystitis and What to Do About It*. Health Education Council, Oxford Street, London.

Kilmartin, Angela. 1973. *Understanding Cystitis*. Hamlyn, London.

Kilmartin, Angela. 1980. *Cystitis: A Complete Self-Help Guide*. Hamlyn, London.

Walton, J. for Nuffield Working Party. 1978. *Talking with Patients: A Teaching Approach*. Observations of a Nuffield Working Party on communications with patients. Nuffield Provincial Hospitals Trust, London.

ADDITIONAL REFERENCES

Watson, J.E. and Royle, J. R. 1987. *Watson's Medical-Surgical Nursing and Related Physiology*, 3rd edition. Baillière Tindall, London.

ANGELA POOLE

Angela finds a lump in her breast and seeks treatment.

Breast cancer is the most common form of cancer in women and presently affects one in seventeen. Treatments include surgery, radiotherapy and drug therapy, all of which present women with potential problems of a physical, emotional and social nature.

As a student you will probably have nursed women with breast cancer.

Try to recall specific patients you have cared for; the difficulties they encountered and overcame.

CHECK ▶ Make sure you understand and investigate the following before completing the study questions in this vignette (see key references on page 180 for useful reading):

1 ▶ The principles of nursing a woman having part or all of her breast removed (mastectomy).

2 ▶ The information which needs to be given to a woman having radiotherapy following breast surgery.

Angela Poole is 52 years old, unmarried, and the headmistress of a village school. She is one of the world's great enthusiasts. Apart from a full working life, she also has a wide-ranging involvement in village activities. As a member of the Church she is the principal organizer of fetes and bazaars, and she works with the Girl Guides and takes them camping two or three times a year. She is an active member of the Golf Club and one of a group of friends who meet to socialize and to play bridge each week. She finds time to tend her garden and grows and freezes practically all the vegetables and fruit she needs.

Like many women, she found the lump in her left breast accidentally whilst in the shower. With her usual 'better get this sorted out' approach, she immediately visited her friend Marjorie, a community nurse, who subsequently arranged an appointment for

Angela with her GP the next morning. Five days later Angela was admitted to hospital in Bristol for investigations and a biopsy of her breast lump.

Angela's surgery, planned for the day after admission to hospital, will establish whether the lump is cancer, and whether it has spread. The lump and the lymph nodes in her axilla will be biopsied and analysed. Once Angela has undergone other investigations to see if, for example, the cancer has spread to her bones or liver (detected by means of bone and liver scans) it will be time for decisions to be made about the treatment she needs.

The treatment of breast cancer, i.e. the extent of surgery, the type of radiotherapy, the use of cytotoxic drugs and the alteration of the hormone balance in the body by surgery or drugs, is being critically scrutinized by doctors, patients and interested members of the public. Some of the areas being analysed are explored in Baum 1981, Kingman 1986 and Alderman 1986.

Although Angela appears to be composed and calm she tells you, on the evening before her biopsy, that she feels she has let herself down a bit over finding the lump, because she has never seriously accepted and practised the habit of examining her breasts in a systematic manner each month. She explains that, even though she went to a talk given by a health visitor in the village some years before when the audience were advised to carry out this regular examination, she had not been convinced sufficiently to practise it.

In some nursing textbooks nurses, in their role as health educators, are expected to teach women to practise breast self-examination (BSE). Yet the value of BSE is questioned for a number of reasons. A brief summary of the arguments is given in Holmes 1987.

Another form of screening, that of mammography, is being instituted. For a discussion of this see Sadler 1987.

Angela has the biopsy and undergoes bone and liver scans. She is discharged from hospital and given an out-patient appointment for two weeks later.

1   Investigate what happens in brain, bone and liver scans using radioactive isotopes.
2   When the opportunity arises, go along with a patient undergoing these tests. Try to develop your knowledge of the specific information that a patient needs to know beforehand about the test and what they might experience. Ask patients about the physical sensations they experience during such tests. Add to this information that which is commonly reported to technicians who carry out the tests. (See Manning and McCready 1978, Becher and Maisey 1981a, b.)

TWO WEEKS LATER

Angela Poole is readmitted to a surgical ward. She is to undergo surgery to remove the cancer and to remove the axillary lymph nodes. Following the surgery a course of radiotherapy is to be given.

Write an outline of the specific pre-operative preparation Angela will need, taking into account the information you have gathered so far. (See Wilson-Barnett 1981, Webb 1983, Tschudin 1983; and for mastectomy see Nichols 1981 and Tierney 1984.)

At this point Angela meets for the second time the clinical nurse specialist, Celia Lewis, who is involved with the care of patients with breast cancer (see Gavin 1985 for an account of this job). On this occasion Celia is able to be more specific about the information she can give Angela. They explore what the surgery and radiotherapy will involve, and how Celia will see Angela in the out-patient department over the next few months.

Angela has her operation and appears to recover well from it. She practises her arm exercises. The wound heals, the surgical clips are removed and she is ready for discharge home. One of her most welcome visitors during the final few days before discharge is a member of the Mastectomy Association.

This association, with its volunteer helpers who have experienced mastectomy themselves, is an important example of the associations which have developed in order to meet the needs of people with specific health problems, such as various forms of cancer.

Find out which voluntary associations and self-help groups can be offered to women with breast cancer, and to cancer patients generally, in your local area.

FOLLOWING DISCHARGE FROM HOSPITAL

When Celia Lewis sees Angela during her course of radiotherapy treatment and at her out-patient clinic appointments, she attempts to assess Angela physically, psychologically and socially, and tries to maintain and build up the relationship between herself and Angela. Angela is able to contact her by telephone in between her clinic visits if she needs assistance. (The need for continued counselling and support for mastectomy patients is explored in Maguire 1978 and Cox 1984.)

DISCUSSION AND FURTHER STUDY

Angela wished to return to her previous way of life. She chose to explain truthfully to her friends about her health problems and she continues to have their support and friendship in her many social activities.

1   Breast cancer, after initial treatment with combinations of surgery, radiotherapy and chemotherapy, can recur. Women may experience bouts of physical ill health, with, for example, bone pain and fracture and symptoms of hypercalcaemia if they have bone metastases. The ability to cope with the symptoms of metastatic breast disease is discussed in McLean 1986 and Batehup 1986.

2   Breast cancer can be treated in a number of ways. Sometimes radiotherapy is used as the principal treatment rather than surgery. One method is to treat the cancer with ionizing radiation from radioactive irridium wires temporarily implanted in the breast. See Jones 1984.

   Breast cancer metastasizes early in its natural history and cytotoxic drugs may be used to eradicate these metastases. For details see Taylor 1984.

3   In 1987 the government accepted the recommendations of a report of a working group chaired by Sir Patrick Forrest which looked into screening for breast cancer. The report is reviewed in Sadler 1987.

   What is being done by your Health Authority to translate government policy and the Report's recommendations into practice?

4   Try to organize the opportunity in a study block to practise role-playing the situation between Angela and her nurse when she expresses concern that she has 'let herself down' by not examining her breasts regularly. Role-playing should be done with the assistance of a teacher or someone experienced in using it. It can leave you in a state of emotional turmoil unless the session is carefully brought to a close. If you are unable to organize a role-playing session you can instead think through, on your own, what you might say in response to Angela's questions.

5   Other situations which can be examined by role-play, or by thinking through what you would say, include:
   (a)   the patient who asks you if you would go ahead with the treatment for breast cancer that her doctor is proposing;
   (b)   the patient who asks you if taking the contraceptive pill and smoking has caused her to develop cancer.

REFERENCES TO VIGNETTE 15

KEY REFERENCES

Marks-Maran, D. J. and Pope, B. M. 1985. *Breast Cancer Nursing and Counselling*. Blackwell Scientific Publications, London.

Tiffany, R. (ed.) 1978. *Oncology for Nurses and Health Care Professionals. Volume I. Pathology, Diagnosis and Treatment*. George Allen & Unwin, London.

Tiffany, R. (ed.) 1980. *Cancer Nursing. Surgical*. Faber & Faber, London.

Webb, C. 1985. *Sexuality, Nursing and Health*. John Wiley & Sons, London.

ADDITIONAL REFERENCES

Alderman, C. 1986. A woman's right to choose. *Nursing Times*, 15 October, pp.18–19.

Batehup, L. 1986. Relieving pain for a patient with breast cancer. *Nursing Times*, 19 November, pp. 36–9.

Baum, M. 1981. *Breast Cancer. The Facts.* Oxford University Press, Oxford.

Becher, C. and Maisey, M. 1981a. Nuclear medicine and nursing. I: Tracing disease to its source. *Nursing Mirror*, 26 August, pp. 16–17.

Becher, C. and Maisey, M. 1981b. Nuclear medicine and nursing. II: A picture of health? Radioisotopes in diagnostic technique. *Nursing Mirror*, 2 September, pp.34–6.

Cox, E. 1984. Psychological aspects. *Nursing Mirror*, 14 November, pp.18–19.

Gavin, A. 1985. Patience first. *Senior Nurse*, 13 February, pp.16–18.

Holmes, P. 1987. Examining the evidence. *Nursing Times*, 5 August, pp.28–30.

Jones, J. 1984. Breast cancer 2: Nursing care study. Primary radiotherapy. *Nursing Mirror*, 21 November, pp.34, 36.

Kingman, S. 1986. Consensus on breast cancer. *New Scientist*, 112, 13 November, pp. 48–51.

McLean, G. 1986. One day at a time. *Nursing Times*, 3 September, pp. 28–31.

Maguire, G. P. 1978. The psychological effects of cancers and their treatments. In Tiffany, R. (ed.) above.

Manning, D. J. and McCready, V. R. 1978. Radioisotope imaging in oncology. In Tiffany, R. (ed.) above.

Nichols, S. 1981. Mastectomy personal experience – breast cancer. *Nursing Mirror*, 11 November, pp.46–8.

Sadler, C. 1987. The breast report. *Nursing Times*, 7 October, pp.31–2.

Taylor, A. 1984. Breast cancer I: Medical treatment. *Nursing Mirror*, 14 November, pp.16–17.

Tierney, J. 1984. Breast cancer I: 'Breast off'. *Nursing Mirror*, 14 November, pp.20–2.

Tschudin, V. 1983. Nursing care study. A quiet confidence. *Nursing Times*, 26 January, pp.32–5.

Webb, C. 1983. Teaching for recovery from surgery. In Wilson-Barnett, J. (ed.) *Patient Teaching*. Churchill Livingstone, Edinburgh.

Wilson-Barnett, J. 1981. Keeping patients informed. *Nursing*, 1st series, 31 November, pp.1357–8.

SAMANTHA RICE

Samantha, aged 4½, has acute leukaemia.

Children with leukaemia and their families have prolonged contact with health care professionals in clinics and hospital wards. The care we give as nurses is therefore directed towards supporting and helping to sustain the child and all his or her family through situations 'good' and 'bad'.

Nursing children who have a life-threatening illness and caring for their families can be an experience through which we learn much.

Recall the paediatric ward you worked in and your experiences with severely ill children. What important things did you learn?

If you have not yet nursed in a paediatric ward, bring to mind the sort of concerns you have right now about this aspect of nursing.

CHECK ▶	Make sure you understand and investigate the following before completing the study questions in this vignette (see key references on page 186 for useful literature):

1 ▶   The function of the bone marrow, red blood cells, white blood cells and platelets.

2 ▶   The pathology and treatment of leukaemia, in adults and children.

Samantha Rice is a lively four-year-old child with a brother Mark, nine years old, and a sister Jeanette who is seven. Margaret Rice, her mother, noticed, over a period of two months, that Sammy seemed quieter than usual and was less active.

Margaret took her daughter to her family doctor when Sammy developed a throat infection, and at the same time bruises on her skin and bleeding from her gums when she brushed her teeth.

Sammy was admitted to hospital where a diagnosis of acute lymphoblastic leukaemia was made. Her care was then taken over by a paediatrician in Manchester, twenty-six miles away, and she was admitted to a children's ward there.

Given the background information you have so far, and taking into account your knowledge about the needs of a four-year-old child, what do you feel should be the most important goals a nurse should try to achieve with Sammy and her mother by the end of her first day on the ward?

The needs of children in hospital is reported in Hawthorn 1974. Look at this piece of research and consider its findings. (See also Rodin 1983.)

An important feature of caring for children in hospital is that staff try to enable parents to be with their children as much as possible. This will help to lessen their anxiety about being in unfamiliar surroundings and undergoing often unpleasant sensations. Thus for this particular family Mrs Rice has decided to stay with her sister who lives in Manchester. This will mean that she can be with Sammy in the ward for most of the time. Back home, Mark and Jeanette are cared for by Colin Rice's mother and himself.

In order to control the leukaemia, Sammy is to be treated with intravenous cytotoxic drugs. She will probably require intravenous infusions of blood and specific blood products such as platelets and white blood cells and will need to have blood samples taken, sometimes daily, to monitor the progress of her treatment. She has already experienced blood tests and a bone marrow aspiration, all of which involved 'needles', and Sammy is already scared of them and the pain they bring.

Like other children in her situation, Sammy had a central venous line, a Hickman catheter, inserted whilst she had a general anaesthetic. This is used to give her treatment and will mean that she will have injections and contact with needles only occasionally.

You may have cared for patients with Hickman catheters already. There are usually specific guidelines for caring for patients with such catheters in each hospital. A brief outline is given in Hollingsworth 1987.

Samantha, at four years old, is developing physically, socially and intellectually. She is acquiring greater abilities in motor skills – walking, running and climbing, and in painting and using pencils. She is able to use words with greater skill. At this stage she feels safe with her parents and siblings but is also able to develop relationships with other children and begins to be able to play co-operatively with them.

Knowledge about a child's intellectual, social and physical skills will influence the way in which they are nursed. For a full discussion of the developmental level of a child like Samantha see Bee, H., 1981. *The developing child*, 3rd edition. Harper & Row, New York.

Check with your teacher and librarian about other resources.

Sammy is going to be treated with cytotoxic drugs in order to control and hopefully cure the leukaemia.

Cytotoxic drug therapy is used in the treatment of cancer in adults and children.

1   What is the action of these drugs, and how is it usefully harnessed in the treatment of cancer?

2   Investigate the unwanted effects (side-effects) of the following cytotoxic drugs which can be used at different stages in the treatment of leukaemia:

vincristine;

cytosine arabinoside;

methotrexate;

daunarubicin.

3   Investigate what care given by nurses and patients will be needed in order to minimize and ameliorate the discomfort of the side effects of the drug treatment.

(See Becker 1981, Holmes 1986a, b.)

In addition to being nursed by her mother, Samantha has her very 'own' nurse, Liza Stevens. Nursing in the children's ward is managed by means of a primary nursing system and this prolonged contact between nurse, child and family has meant that Liza has been able to become knowledgeable and skilful in nursing Sammy and in supporting her mother. (For further information on primary nursing, see page 33; also read Geen 1986.)

Samantha achieves 'remission' six weeks later, with the cytotoxic drug treatment and does not experience physiological crises such as haemorrhage because of insufficient platelets, or widespread infection because of insufficient white blood cells.

However, whilst undergoing cytotoxic drug treatment she does become neutropaenic. She is nursed in a single room and because of her susceptibility to infection is 'reverse barrier nursed'.

Whilst undergoing treatment Sammy has insufficient white blood cells to overcome infection and so great care is taken to prevent her becoming infected.

The main source of microorganisms causing infection is herself, those inside and on her body which can cause problems. For a discussion about the care of the neutropaenic patient and reverse barrier nursing refer to your hospital's nursing procedure book or:

Royal Marsden Hospital. 1984. *Manual of clinical nursing policies and procedures.* Chapter 3. Lippincott Nursing Series. Harper and Row. London.

One area that becomes infected and causes discomfort is the mouth – so mouth hygiene is very important. For a discussion of this see Campbell 1987.

Sammy is soon discharged home, and returns each week for further monitoring of her disease and cytotoxic drug treatment. She will also undergo some radiotherapy to her cranium to destroy leukaemic cells there. On each visit she returns to the ward to see Liza and have her treatment.

Treatments for leukaemia do vary over time and from hospital to hospital.

1   Find out the treatment 'protocols' for leukaemia in your district. The protocol will vary according to the type of leukaemia and the age of the person concerned.

2   Nurses have written about the care and long-term treatment of children with leukaemia in Robotham 1983, Flockhart 1983 and Richards 1985.

Samantha's parents, Margaret and Colin, are also given support by Liza and the other staff involved in Sammy's care. As parents they face the distress of having a child with a potentially fatal illness, one which involves continuous treatment and monitoring. They know the leukaemic process may return and Sammy may need further treatment. In addition, they have to face the task of trying to maintain as normal a family life as is possible for their two other children.

What resources and which people in the community are available for parents like Margaret and Colin?

DISCUSSION AND FURTHER STUDY

During the period of remission, Sammy's parents may need to decide whether or not to agree to a bone-marrow transplant. This will bring the prospect of long-term cure but it is also traumatic, distressing and can fail.

1   Try to investigate the topic of bone-marrow transplants. The experiences of a nurse undergoing a transplant is given in Gibson, L. 1987. Bone-marrow transplant – the process. *Nursing Times.* 21 January, pp.36–8.

2   In this vignette we have looked at leukaemia in a child. Investigate the differences in treatment for adults, and for chronic leukaemia in contrast to acute forms of leukaemia.

3   There has been public concern expressed about the incidence of leukaemia in areas with nuclear establishments. Become aware of this and develop your own information file. Try to evaluate the different perspectives and possible bias shown within different journals, newspapers and in the broadcast media about this subject. (See Darby and Doll 1987.)

4   Specialist nursing journals are available in the field of cancer nursing and will detail practice and research in this developing area in nursing. Both are published in the United States: *Cancer nursing* and *Oncology Nursing Forum.*

REFERENCES TO VIGNETTE 16

KEY REFERENCES

Lakhani, A. K. 1987. Current management of acute leukaemia. *Nursing*, 3rd series, No.20, pp.755–8.

Nursing Mirror Supplement. 1980. Childhood cancer. *Nursing Mirror*, 28 August.

Maguire, P. 1978. The psychological effects of cancers and their treatments. In Tiffany, R. (ed.) *Oncology for Nurses and Health Care Professionals*, Vol.2. Allen & Unwin, London.

Tiffany, R. (ed.) 1978 *Oncology for Nurses and Health Care Professionals. Vol.I: Pathology, Diagnosis and Treatment.* Allen & Unwin, London.

Tiffany, R. (ed.) 1979. *Cancer Nursing. Medical.* Faber & Faber, London.

ADDITIONAL REFERENCES

Becker, T. M. 1981. *Cancer Chemotherapy: A Manual for Nurses.* Little, Brown, Boston.

Campbell, S. 1987. Mouthcare in cancer patients. *Nursing Times*, 22 July, pp.59–60.

Darby, S. C. and Doll, R. 1987. Fallout, radiation doses near Dounreay and childhood leukaemia. *British Medical Journal*, 294, 7 March, pp.603–7.

Flockhart, J. 1983. A shadow hanging over us. *Nursing Mirror*, 6 April, pp.32–4.

Geen L. 1986. A special friend. *Nursing Times*, 3 September, pp.32–3.

Hawthorn, P. J. 1974. *Nurse, I Want My Mummy!* RCN, London.

Hollingsworth, S. 1987. Getting on line. *Nursing Times*, 22 July, pp.61–2.

Holmes, S. 1986a. Action of cancer chemotherapy. *Professional Nurse*, 2(2), November, pp.45–6.

Holmes, S. 1986b. How to administer chemotherapy. *Professional Nurse*, 2(3), December, pp.72–4.

Richards, I. 1985. Breaking the silence. *Nursing Times*, 30 October, pp.32–5.

Robotham, A. 1983. Children with leukaemia. *Nursing Times*, 16 February, pp.28–9.

Rodin, J. 1983. Preparing children for hospital. In Wilson-Barnett, J. (ed.) *Nursing Research: Ten Studies in Patient Care.* Wiley & Sons, London.

JAMES RYDER

James is admitted to hospital with sickle cell crisis.

There are people with health problems which, in their estimation, do not receive sufficient resources and attention by the professionals and managers of the National Health Service. They feel that their needs are not being met. One such group, it would appear, are those people who have sickle cell trait and sickle cell disease (sickle cell anaemia).

Bring to mind patients you have nursed who were anaemic, particularly those with sickle cell disease.

How did their health problem affect their daily lives?

CHECK ▶ | Make sure you understand and investigate the following before completing the study questions in this vignette (for useful reading, see key references, page 190):

1 ▶ The development of red blood cells in the body.

2 ▶ The incidence of sickle cell disease in the population served by your Health Authority.

James Ryder, aged 25, is a bus driver, and has sickle cell disease (sickle cell anaemia). This is an inherited blood disorder which can affect people like James who are of Afro-Caribbean origin. James is one of the estimated 2000 people in London who live with this health problem.

In this blood disorder the red blood cells are fragile and have a shorter than normal lifespan, and the haemoglobin in the red cells is abnormal. In situations of low oxygen tension (hypoxia) the red cells assume a 'sickle' shape and clump together and block small blood vessels (infarction). This is known as a sickle cell crisis. The organs and tissues distal to the blocked blood vessels become ischaemic, and this results in pain and tissue damage. Although no part of the body is exempt from this process, the bones, spleen, kidneys, gastro-intestinal tract and lungs are most commonly affected.

James is thought to have developed a viral infection in his lungs and this has triggered off this crisis. On admission he is sweating, pyrexial and breathless and has chest pain. He feels exhausted because he has not slept for two nights and he has been feeling very tired and unwell for the past month.

Use the information you have so far about James, and make a list of what you see as the most important aspects of nursing care needed by him on admission to hospital.

One aspect, your main priority, will be pain relief. This will be best achieved by accurately assessing and treating the different pains James has. A pain assessment tool is likely to be helpful in assessing the pain and whether it is being alleviated. James will probably need narcotic analgesia initially, for example, I.M. Pethidine.

Pain assessment and relief by nurses is discussed in Sofaer, 1984 and Gollop 1983. The first edition of *Nursing* (April 1979) is all about pain and pain control.

James tells you there is no 'cure' for his illness but he explains that when he gets symptoms which are mild he sorts them out himself by means of resting, taking pain killers, and drinking plenty of fluids. When the symptoms got too bad and he was admitted to hospital he had been treated with pain relief, rest, and on different occasions oxygen therapy, blood transfusion and intravenous fluids and antibiotics.

At this point you may want to review the knowledge you need in order to plan effective care for someone like James who is having:

1   a blood transfusion;
2   an intravenous infusion to correct dehydration and electrolyte imbalance;
3   oxygen therapy;
4   treatment with intravenous or intramuscular injections of antibiotics.

If you need help, consult the 'procedure book' used in your School of Nursing, a nursing textbook like Watson and Royle (1987) or Roper (1985), or Royal Marsden Hospital 1984.

For a discussion of the equipment used in oxygen therapy, see Levi 1979.

During the evening, James's brother Lennox comes in with his girl friend Lois. Lois is pregnant, and towards the end of visiting time she comes up to you and asks you to help her with something.

How will you deal with this request from a visitor? Write down the principal points of the strategy you would use.

Your strategy in this situation will include at least the following: acknowledging and accepting that she is distressed and has a problem. If you can find a quiet place, you can allow her to talk and can give her encouragement by asking open questions.

Lois explains that she is worried about the health of her baby. She had not realized until recently that Lennox' brother had sickle cell disease and someone at work has told her that her baby may also have it because it runs in families. (Potential sources of information about screening and counselling in sickle cell trait and disease are to be found in Anionwu and Beattie 1981, and Anionwu 1983.)

In responding to Lois's request for advice you could give information yourself and also suggest she talks with her midwife at her next antenatal visit. In the meantime she could also request information from her local Community Health Council, Citizens Advice Bureau or Health Education Authority office. She could also contact the advisers at the Sickle Cell Society.

If a person has sickle cell disease or sickle cell trait this may effect children that they conceive with partners who may have the disease or carry the trait. It seems that Lennox and Lois do not know if they are affected. This lack of awareness on their part may be the direct result of not being screened themselves at birth for the trait or the disease.

In Merry France-Dawson's article (1986) she refers to evidence that sickle cell disease and trait are statistically more common than phenylketonuria and hypothyroidism, both of which are routinely screened for in the newborn in the United Kingdom. However, at the time she writes only 6 out of 76 District Health Authorities with ethnic minority populations of over 3% had any provision for screening for sickle cell trait and disease.

Why may this situation have arisen? (See also Prashar 1985.)

James recovers from the crisis and is discharged from hospital after a few days. He is both knowledgeable about, and capable of maintaining, his health. If he were not it would be essential to ensure he was given information about his health problem and helped and supported in making decisions and choices about the changes in life-style he may need to make.

People with sickle cell disease try, where possible, to prevent acute crises occurring. Bearing in mind the factors which can trigger such crises, outline for yourself the points to be included on a teaching plan that:

1   a hospital nurse, a health visitor or a school nurse would use in teaching parents of a child with sickle cell disease (see Upton 1983).

2   a hospital nurse would use with a person experiencing a sickle cell crisis for the first time;

3   a midwife with a pregnant woman with sickle cell disease and a newly delivered mother whose baby has sickle cell trait.

**DISCUSSION AND
FURTHER STUDY**

In this vignette we have looked at the care of a person with a health problem that occurs in a specific group in society. It is essentially a health problem that requires a person to maintain their health and well-being within the constraints of having a chronic condition which may 'flare up' from time to time. Care given during crises is focused on managing symptoms, the principal one being pain.

In completing this vignette you may like to go on to study further.

1   Develop your knowledge of Afro-Caribbean culture and consider the implications for nursing.

2   How does your Health Authority meet the specific needs of people from ethnic minority groups in your local area. The Health Authority's Strategic Plan for the next five or ten years may be a useful resource and your librarian or a senior nursing manager may be able to assist.

3   Sickle cell anaemia is caused by an abnormality of the haemoglobin molecule. Other forms of anaemia are caused in part by other shortcomings of the red blood cells, their system of production and destruction, and failure of the bone marrow. Make sure you can outline the causes, effects and treatment of other anaemias which people develop:
        iron deficiency anaemia;
        aplastic anaemia;
        pernicious anaemia;
        haemolytic anaemia.

4   Attempt to analyse the following situation and pinpoint the ethical issues involved:

        Joan Tyson is 23 and expecting her second baby. You meet her whilst undertaking your obstetric placement. Listening to the assessment interview between Joan and her midwife at the clinic, you hear her respond that as far as she knows she has no health problems and answers that she does not have sickle cell disease or trait. On examining her medical records you see a haematology report which has 'sickle cell trait' stamped on it.

REFERENCES TO VIGNETTE 17

KEY REFERENCES

Faulkner, A. 1985. *Nursing. A Creative Approach*. Baillière Tindall, London.

France-Dawson, M. 1986. Sickle cell disease: Implications for nursing care. *Journal of Advanced Nursing*, II(6), November, pp.729–37.

Houston, J. C., Joiner, C. L. and Trounce, J. R. 1982. *A Short Textbook of Medicine*, 7th edition. Hodder & Stoughton, London.

Watson, J. E. and Royle, J. R. 1987. *Watson's Medical-Surgical Nursing and Related Physiology*, 3rd edition. Baillière Tindall, London.

Wilson, K. J. W. 1987. *Ross and Wilson. Anatomy and Physiology in Health and Illness*, 6th edition. Churchill Livingstone, Edinburgh.

ADDITIONAL REFERENCES

Anionwu, E. N. 1983. Sickle cell disease: screening and counselling in the antenatal and neonatal period. *Midwife Health Visitor and Community Nurse*, Part I: October, pp.402, 404, 406. Part 2: November, pp.440–3.

Anionwu, E. M. and Beattie, A. 1981. Learning to cope with sickle cell disease – a parent's experience. *Nursing Times*, 8 July, pp.1214–19.

Gollop, S. M. 1983. *Patient Teaching: Pain and Pain Control*. In Wilson-Barnett, J. (ed.) *Patient Teaching*. Churchill Livingstone, Edinburgh.

Levi, T. 1979. Breathing equipment. *Nursing*, Part I, 1st series. 6 September, pp.206–3 and 7 November, pp.336–9.

Prashar, U. 1985. The disease that discriminates. *Nursing Times*, 4 September, pp.16–17.

Royal Marsden Hospital. 1984. *Manual of Clinical Nursing Policies and Procedures*. Harper & Row, London.

Sofaer, B. 1984. *Pain: A Handbook for Nurses*. Lippincott Nursing series. Harper & Row, London.

Upton, M. 1983. Nursing care study. Young Winston. *Nursing Mirror*, 10 August, pp.46–8.

MAVIS SNOWDEN

Mavis experiences a profound change in body image because of an endocrine disorder.

In this vignette we consider the problems which can arise when the hormonal balance in the body is disrupted. Although this is due to malfunction of the adrenal glands, some of the effects on the body of the person affected will remind you of the side-effects of steroid drugs.

Recall patients you have nursed who have either Cushing's Syndrome or have experienced the side-effects of steroid drugs.

How was their health affected?

CHECK ▶

Make sure you understand and investigate the following before completing the study questions in this vignette (see key references, page 196, for useful reading):

1 ▶ Revise the physiology of the endocrine system, and take particular note of the functioning of the adrenal glands.

2 ▶ Investigate the unwanted effects of steroid drugs and compare them with the physiological effects of Cushing's Syndrome.

3 ▶ Consider the concept of sexuality and its significance in nursing practice.

Mavis Snowden, aged 45, is sitting in the day-room of a ward at a District General Hospital. She feels awkward and self-conscious. The trouble is that she has become a changed woman over the last two years.

From your background reading about Cushing's Syndrome, list the effects that it will have had on Mrs Snowden's body.

Try at the same time to relate the changes experienced to the underlying physiology of this disorder.

Mrs Snowden feels depressed and unhappy much of the time. She keeps remembering ten years ago when she was a manageress at the Crown and Eagle hotel in the High Street. She had been popular with everyone, and she found herself being 'chatted up' by many of the customers when she supervised things in the cocktail bar and the coffee lounge. She had always taken pleasure in looking after her skin and hair, and in wearing fashionable clothes.

But recently she found herself so changed by her illness that she no longer has the confidence to go for part-time jobs. She feels tired all the time and tries to get a good night's sleep by going to bed early and yet she never does. She has gained a great deal of weight and is horrified by the condition of her skin, the acne, and the growth of hair on her face.

It was her daughter, June, who made Mavis go to see her general practitioner. Mavis found him to be very helpful and sympathetic. He said that the changes in her appearance indicated that she had a problem with her 'glands and hormones'. Mavis was admitted to the endocrinology ward of the hospital where she underwent numerous blood and urine tests, and a CT scan which showed that her right adrenal gland was enlarged. She has now been admitted to hospital for surgical removal of the adrenal gland and hopefully resolution of her health problem.

Look up the concept of body-image or self-image in Webb 1985 and Lion 1982.

In what way will a knowledge of human sexuality help us to nurse patients like Mrs Snowden?

By now you have a picture of Mrs Snowden as a person who has undergone a profound change in the appearance of her body and also in its functioning.

Here is the nursing assessment recorded for Mrs Snowden:

◊ *Maintaining a safe environment*
Bones may be affected by osteoporosis, therefore prone to fractures. Tendency to bruise easily.

◊ *Communicating*
Says she feels depressed. Did talk about her situation and was able to voice some of her feelings about her appearance. Did express a wish to start enployment again when 'all this is sorted out'.

◊ *Breathing*
Gets breathless on exertion ?due to obesity. Doesn't smoke. Chest X-ray normal.

◊ *Eating and drinking*
Weight 100kg. Height 162cms. Obese, with fat distribution pattern normal for a person with Cushing's Syndrome. Feels

hungry most of the time. Eats large helpings at mealtimes and biscuits and snacks throughout the day. Drinks about ten cups of sweetened tea or coffee and cans of soft drink throughout the day.

◊   *Elimination*

Has symptoms of cystitis, and her vulval area feels sore. She has glycosuria. Bowels – a tendency towards passing constipated stools – possibly due to diet – relatively little roughage although plenty of fluids are taken.

◊   *Personal cleansing and dressing*

Enjoys having a bath but finds difficulty with getting out of her bath at home therefore uses shower spray. Does not remove facial hair, 'can't be bothered', and has neglected hairstyling for the past six months; hair held back with elastic band in a ponytail.

◊   *Maintaining body temperature*

Normal temperature – need to observe for pyrexia and possible infection.

◊   *Mobilizing*

Feels very self-conscious when she goes out shopping so does not choose to go out unless she absolutely has to. Has never really been keen on outdoor activities or sports. Able to walk around safely.

◊   *Working and playing*

Watches daytime television and reads library books. Has been unable to get employment. Sometimes knits garments for friends. Financial situation – is supported by mother and social security payments.

◊   *Expressing sexuality*

Very aware of her appearance. Feels she looks 'awful'. Is shutting herself away at home because she feels she has no alternative. Avoids meeting men.

◊   *Sleeping*

Mrs Snowden has difficulty with sleeping – she finds it difficult to get to sleep and wakes early. She doesn't feel rested at the end of the night. But often dozes off in a chair at home during the afternoon.

◊   *Dying*

Feels pretty hopeless at present and wishes she had some zest for life again.

Temperature 37^4

Blood pressure $\frac{155}{85}$

Urinalysis: has glycosuria

Given the information you have about Mrs Snowden, try to pinpoint the key problems she has which should be focused on whilst she is in hopsital.

Write a care plan, taking into account the information in her nursing assessment and her forthcoming surgery.

Mrs Snowden has adapted to the stress of the changes in her body image by withdrawing from meeting and dealing with strangers, and by eating far in excess of her body's needs, even taking into account her increased appetite as a result of her illness. Her doctor has explained to her that once her 'problem', the adrenal gland, is removed, the changes she has experienced with her appearance will cease.

Given that adrenalectomy will remove the excessive amounts of hormones which have caused Mrs Snowden's body to change, and provided the maintenance doses of steroids which she may need to take following surgery do not cause problems, what health teaching can be given to her about:

(a)   reducing her weight;
(b)   removing facial hair;
(c)   dealing with acne;
(d)   taking long-term medication, specifically steroid drugs;
(e)   making social contact with people again

DISCUSSION AND FURTHER STUDY

In this vignette we have considered one cause of a change in the functioning of the body which results in changes in a person's appearance. These changes affect the way a person then feels about herself. Mrs Snowden, for example, felt unattractive and had lost confidence in herself.

The surgery she underwent required careful post-operative nursing (as outlined in Jones 1982). Thoughtful supportive health education by nurses was also needed to help her feel able to take control again over her appearance.

Extend your study notes by investigating:

1   (a)   Under-secretion of the adrenal glands which occurs in Addison's disease. Consider the way this disorder will affect patients.

    (b)   Over- and under-secretion of other endocrine glands, particularly the thyroid.

2   Other vignettes which address the topic of sexuality are Angela Poole with breast cancer, Peter Gray with AIDS. Another vignette which considers endocrine disorders is that about Derek Williams, who has diabetes mellitus.

REFERENCES TO VIGNETTE 18

KEY REFERENCES

Jones, S. G. 1982. Adrenal patient: proceed with caution. *R.N.* 45(1), January, pp.67–8, 70, 72. (This is an American journal; your librarian may be able to obtain a copy for you.

Lion, E. M. (ed.) 1982. *Human Sexuality in Nursing Process.* John Wiley & Sons, New York.

Maxwell, M. 1983. The endocrine system. *Nursing Mirror*, 3 August, pp.23–8.

Millward, E. 1983. The adrenal glands. *Nursing*, 2(13), May, pp.380, 382–3.

Webb, C. 1985. *Sexuality, Nursing and Health.* John Wiley & Sons, London.

GEORGE STEVENS

George came into hospital for 'routine' surgery.

Coming into hospital for 'routine' surgery is routine only in that there is a pattern of pre-operative preparation which is completed in order to safeguard the patient. However, having surgery is often a new and alarming experience for patients, one which may have been awaited over a period of time, or one which is unexpected and linked to a sudden episode of ill-health.

Try to recall and then make a list of as many patients having surgery whom you have nursed over the past six months.

Go through the list and make a note of the individual needs of these people that you tried to meet when you nursed them.

CHECK ▶

Make sure you understand and investigate the following before completing the study questions in this vignette (see key references, page 200 for useful reading):

1 ▶ The symptoms a person with an inguinal hernia may experience, and the potential complications which may arise in the period before the hernia is repaired by surgery.

2 ▶ The principles underlying the nursing of a patient having surgical repair of an inguinal hernia.

This was the second time in a fortnight that George Stevens had arrived at the admissions desk of his local hospital. This time he did not have to go home again because a bed was available for him. He had been waiting for almost a year now to have surgery to an inguinal hernia.

George was one of the four 'routine' admissions on Argos Ward that morning. He sat with three other patients outside the ward. The ward receptionist organized cups of tea and coffee for them and checked the information on the nursing record sheets. Mr Stevens will have surgery the next morning and then, provided he recovers well from the surgery and the general anaesthetic, he will be discharged home in about five days.

Nurses on this surgical ward use standard pre-operative care plans for patients having hernia repairs. These care plans have printed on them the usual goals of care for such patients and the nursing activities needed to meet those goals. There is space to record when the standard care activities have been done, and each patient's individual needs and the care planned to meet them.

Write a list of the goals of care for a patient having a repair of an inguinal hernia, and the nursing activities to meet them. In other words write out a standard pre-operative care plan for these patients. If you are not used to using standard care plans, an example is given on p.121 of Faulkner, A. 1985. *Nursing. A Creative Approach.* Baillière Tindall. London.

You may use pre-operative checklists in your Health District and the contents of the list will reflect some of the essential care needed by patients before surgery which appears on some standard care plans.

One of the important goals of care for a patient undergoing surgery and general anaesthesia, and indeed any investigation, is to ensure that the patient has been given enough information about the procedure to enable him or her to understand what will happen. This will help him or her to be able to cope.

Investigate some of the nursing research about preparing patients for surgery and investigations. i.e. Wilson-Barnett 1978, 1979, Webb 1983, Hayward 1975, Boore 1978.

Mr Stevens' nursing assessment reveals only one specific individual need – that of a desire to lose weight. The nurse who weighed him on admission noticed he was embarrassed about being weighed and said 'I hope I won't break the scales!', and she explored this further with him. His need to be given information and to be counselled further about losing weight to improve his health was written on his care plan.

During that evening Mr Stevens' operation area was shaved and he was given two glycerine suppositories to empty his rectum. He ate his supper at 6 p.m. and understood that from midnight onwards he was not to eat or drink anything.

The practices of skin preparation, bowel preparation and fasting pre-operatively have been investigated. Critically assess Mr Stevens' care with regard to these three topics:

(a)   skin preparation (Stokes 1984);
(b)   bowel preparation (Peters 1983);
(c)   pre-operative fasting (Hamilton-Smith 1972, Hunt 1987).

Next morning Mr Stevens was prepared for his premedication and his transfer to theatre. His surgery was completed and he recovered from the general anaesthetic and was returned to the ward by lunchtime.

Review at this point the routine pre-operative preparation of patients and their early post-operative care. You may find this information in your School of Nursing's procedure book. (See also Royal Marsden Hospital 1984.)

Mr Stevens' vital signs of temperature, pulse and blood pressure all remained within normal limits in his immediate post-operative period and by the evening he was sitting up in bed, feeling drowsy and slightly nauseated, but otherwise well. He was given I.M. Omnopon 15mg for pain relief and I.M. Prochlorperazine 12.5mg to prevent him vomiting.

Ensuring that patients are not in pain post-operatively is of fundamental importance in nursing practice. Being in pain, apart from causing unnecessary suffering for patients, will prevent them from being able to carry out deep breathing and leg exercises which are necessary to avoid post-operative complications such as chest infection and deep-veined thrombosis (see Seers 1987).

Mr Stevens' wound has been closed with clips and covered with a piece of gauze and a waterpoof top dressing. His dressing is renewed three days after surgery. There is no evidence of infection and Mr Stevens is not experiencing any discomfort.

What are the best conditions for healing to take place? A number of factors are involved, both internal factors within the person, and external factors within the environment. (See Westaby 1981a, b and Jaber 1986.)

Mr Stevens left hospital five days after he had been admitted.

How would you plan for his discharge home?

What information and advice does he need before leaving the ward?

DISCUSSION AND FURTHER STUDY

Mr Stevens has undergone surgery for a health problem which was causing him discomfort. His recovery has been uncomplicated and routine. The ward he was nursed on was a busy surgical ward staffed by student nurses, auxiliaries and trained nurses. Mr Stevens feels he has received first-class treatment; he felt reasured by the efficiency of the service. He found the nurses cheerful and friendly and enjoyed the joking and general banter which went on as they they got on with their many tasks.

1 This vignette has enabled you to take a research-minded approach to the care of a patient undergoing surgery. You may also have found yourself seeking out information about other aspects of this patient's care which were not focused on. One area which is of importance is the communication between patients and nurses in surgical wards. This has been investigated by nurses and an outline of the research is given in Macleod Clark 1983.

2 Cross-infection of patients' wounds occurs in a number of ways, including faulty dressing technique and staff not washing their hands properly or often enough. Consider the following research about this problem: Hunt 1974, Sedgewick 1984, Gidley 1987, Blackmore 1987.

REFERENCES FOR VIGNETTE 19

KEY REFERENCES

Ellison Nash, D. F. 1980. *Principles and Practice of Surgery for Nurses and Allied Professions*, 7th edition. Edward Arnold, London.

Faulkner, A. 1985. *Nursing: A Creative Approach*. Baillière Tindall, London.

ADDITIONAL REFERENCES

Blackmore, M. 1987. Hand-drying methods. *Nursing Times*, 16 September, pp.71–2.

Boore, J. 1978. *A Prescription for Recovery*. RCN, London.

Clark, J. Macleod 1983. Nurse–patient communication: An analysis of conversations from surgical wards. In Wilson-Barnett, J. (ed.) *Nursing Research: Ten Studies in Patient Care*. John Wiley & Sons, London.

Draper, J. 1985. Make the dressing fit the wound. *Nursing Times*, 9 October, pp. 32–5.

Gidley, C. 1987. Now, wash your hands! *Nursing Times*, 22 July, pp.40–2.

Hamilton-Smith, S. 1972. Nil by mouth? *RCN*, London.

Hayward, J. 1975. *Information: A prescription against Pain*. RCN, London.

Hunt, J. 1974. *The Teaching and Practice of Surgical Dressings in Three Hospitals*. Royal College of Nursing, London.

Hunt, M. 1987. The process of translating research findings into nursing practice. *Journal of Advanced Nursing*, 12(1), January, pp.101–10.

Jaber, F. 1986. Charting wound healing. *Nursing Times*, 10 September, pp.24–7.

Peters, D. 1983. Bowel preparation for surgery. *Nursing Times*, 13 July, pp.32–4.

Royal Marsden Hospital. 1984. *Manual of Clinical Nursing Policies and Procedures*. Lippincott Nursing series. Harper & Row, London.

Sedgewick, J. 1984. Hand washing in hospital wards. *Nursing Times*, 16 May, pp.64–7.

Seers, K. 1987. Perceptions of pain. *Nursing Times*, 2 December, pp.37–8.

Stokes, E. 1984. Showering before surgery. Shaving before surgery. *Nursing Times*, 16 May, p.71.

Webb, C. 1983. Teaching for recovery from surgery. In Wilson-Barnett, J. (ed.) *Patient Teaching*. Churchill Livingstone, Edinburgh.

Westaby, S. 1981a. Healing: The normal mechanism, I. *Nursing Times*, 18 November, pp.9–12.

Westaby, S. 1981b. Healing: The normal mechanism, II. *Nursing Times*, 16 December, No. 4, pp.13–16.

Wilson-Barnett, J. 1978. Patient's emotional response to barium X-rays. *Journal of Advanced Nursing*, 3, pp.37–46.

Wilson-Barnett, J. 1979. *Stress in Hospital*. Churchill Livingstone, Edinburgh.

JANE WALTERS

Jane chooses to have her pregnancy terminated.

In the following vignette, we will be considering the needs of a woman who discovers that she has an unplanned pregnancy. Of the options open to her, the woman elects to have the pregnancy terminated.

Before reading any further, try to analyse your own opinions about the termination of a pregnancy. The chapter entitled 'Ethical Dilemmas in Nursing' in this book may help you.

| CHECK ▶ | Make sure you understand and investigate the following before completing the study questions in this vignette: |

1 ▶   The Therapeutic Abortion Act of 1967 (described in most gynaecology nursing books).

2 ▶   Foetal development.

3 ▶   Different methods available for terminating a pregnancy.

See key references at the end of this vignette. There are also a number of action groups who can supply useful information. Some of them are the British Pregnancy Advisory Service; The Let Live Association; The Creation Project (furthers vasectomy as a method of birth control); National Consumer Council; Association of Community Health Councils for England and Wales. You can find out more about these action groups in directories such as *Self-Help and The Patient*, published by the Patients Association, 18 Charing Cross Road, London WC2H 0HR.

Jane Walters is a 39-year-old woman who has been married for fifteen years. She and her husband have two sons aged nine and twelve years. Following the birth of their second son, Jane and Alec Walters decided that their family was complete and Alec had a vasectomy. The Walters are central figures in their local community, Jane is a school governor and Alec is a local councillor.

A brief affair with a neighbour leads to Jane's becoming pregnant.

Using a gynaecology book, consider the options open to Jane at this point. Discuss these options and your feelings about them with colleagues.

It may help you to refer back to one of the thought clarification models described in Chapter 5.

Jane decides to have her pregnancy terminated and this is arranged by her GP within the terms of the 1967 Abortion Act.

Having read the act, decide how Jane's GP may have interpreted the act in order to recommend that Jane has a termination.

It is possible that the GP interpreted the clause which refers to 'involving risk to the mental health of the pregnant woman or any existing children of her family greater than if the pregnancy were terminated'. He would, of course, have needed the support of another doctor, but it may have been decided that the distress caused by this pregnancy would adversely affect the lives of the Walters family.

We have referred to the Therapeutic Abortion Act. What does the term 'abortion' mean, and what other types of abortion are there?

You will see that the term 'abortion' refers to any pregnancy which ends before 28 weeks duration. It is very important to understand that many abortions are spontaneous and occur without any intervention. In fact, the lay term 'miscarriage' is interchangeable with the medical term 'spontaneous abortion'. A therapeutic abortion is, you will find, sometimes referred to in hospital as a termination of pregnancy.

Jane Walters is admitted to hospital for the termination of an eight-week pregnancy. This is to be achieved by dilation of the cervix and suction removal of the products of conception.

Again, consult your gynaecology nursing books to gain an understanding of this term.

What other methods may be used to terminate a pregnancy?

Why do you think this was the chosen method for Jane?

If you read a description of foetal development, you will realize that an eight-week foetus is still quite small (about 1¼ inches long and 1/30 ounce in weight). At this stage, then, it is possible to remove the foetus through the vagina despite the fact that this is a very active and crucial period of development.

On admission, Jane is adamant that her husband should not know the real reason for her admission. She has told him that she is to undergo investigations for menstrual disorders.

Does Alec have any right to know the truth?

Does the child's father have any right to prevent the termination?

You could discuss these questions from the legal and the ethical points of view. A useful reference here is A. P. Young, *Legal problems in nursing practice*. (Harper & Row 1981).

The leaflet entitled 'Patients' Rights' produced by the National Consumer Council in conjunction with the Association of Community Health Councils makes the following statement in relation to consent for abortion: 'For an abortion, your consent (the woman's) alone is needed, although doctors might want to consult your partner if you are willing.' In other words, legally the mother can have a pregnancy terminated without reference to the father.

Morally there is, again, no right answer but it is a point which you may like to discuss with your colleagues.

Refer back to the 1967 Act:
What right do nurses and doctors have with regard to therapeutic abortions? Can they refuse to take part in the procedure itself? Can they refuse to care for women who have undergone, or are about to undergo, a termination of pregnancy?

The 1967 Act states that a nurse or doctor can refuse to take part in the actual procedure which results in the termination of a pregnancy. No reference, however, is made to the related care which a woman will require. Nurses have the same human rights as everyone else, so they have the right to refuse to care for a particular patient. However, in making such a decision they would need to be aware of the consequences and these could, in some districts, prove to be fairly drastic. This is a clear example of conflicting rights which may be clarified by the use of Curtin's or Bergman's model (see chapter 5).

Jane undergoes surgery as planned and the pregnancy is terminated.

Are there any specific problems or potential post-operative problems which nursing intervention may prevent or minimize?

Specific immediate post-operative care should be aimed at the detection and monitoring of post-operative haemorrhage.

Once Jane has become alert following the operation, her initial reaction may be one of relief that her ordeal is over and she no longer needs to worry about being pregnant. She may also feel guilty and experience a sense of loss for the child which she is no longer going to have.

Before she is discharged home, it may help Jane to talk to someone about her feelings. She has solved one problem, but it is quite possible that she will experience feelings of grief. Some health districts employ counsellors especially to help women who have undergone a therapeutic termination of pregnancy. Perhaps you know of one in your district.

It may be that Jane has a need of further family planning advice. This could be a sensitive subject, and perhaps simply ensuring that she knows the address of the local clinic will be all you can hope to achieve. Certainly, Jane should be advised to contact her GP if she experiences any secondary haemorrhage or prolonged post-operative bleeding.

FURTHER DISCUSSION

Do you know of any cultures where terminating a pregnancy would not be considered as a possible option? Your most useful resource here may be leaflets produced by the Health Education Authority. Your local Community Health Council may have its own publications and health centres often have leaflets which pertain to the immediate population.

You may find, for example, that within the Sikh culture there is a strong code of sexual morality. Pre-marital and extra-marital sex are forbidden and illicit liaisons bring deep shame upon the family. It is unlikely that a Sikh woman would find herself in Jane's situation. Abortion is generally disapproved of although the deep shame of being unmarried and pregnant may, for example, lead a Sikh woman to consider undergoing a termination of pregnancy.

Bangladeshi girls are raised in a restrictive environment, and their culture dictates that a girl must be a virgin on her marriage, so again it is unlikely that many young Bangladeshi girls will seek termination of a pregnancy.

Rastafarian women would see therapeutic abortion as murder, unnatural and ungodly. In fact, they do not practise birth control as they consider this a form of genocide.

Muslims believe abortion to be very wrong except where it is necessary to save the life of the mother. Very special care is needed for Muslim women who have had a pregnancy terminated, whether it be for medical reasons or without their families knowledge, as both have been done against their faith.

There are just a few examples and you may be able to identify some more.

REFERENCES TO VIGNETTE 20

KEY REFERENCES

Annis, Ferril. 1978. *The Child Before Birth*, ch.1. Cornell University Press, Ithaca, New York.

Bailey, R. E. 1983. *Obstetrics and Gynaecology for Nurses*. Nurses Aids series, Baillière Tindall, London.

Cheetham, Juliet. 1978. *Unwanted Pregnancy and Counselling*. Routledge & Kegan Paul, London.

Clayton, Sir S. and Newton J. 1983. *A Pocket Gynaecology*. Churchill Livingstone, Edinburgh.

Fletcher, J. 1979. *Morals and Medicine*. Princeton University Press, N.J.

Harmon, Vera M. and Steele, S. M. 1983. *Values Clarification in Nursing*. Appleton-Century-Crofts, New York.

Medical Defence Union. 1967. *Memoranda on the Abortion Act 1967 and the Abortion Regulation 1986*. Medical Defence Union, London.

Simmons, W. 1985. *Learning to Care on the Gynaecology Ward*, ch.6. Hodder & Stoughton, London.

Tunnadine, D. and Greene, R. 1978. *Unwanted Pregnancy : Accident or Illness*. Oxford University Press, Oxford.

WILLIAM WATSON AND GRAHAM DAWSON

William and Graham are both admitted to a cardiac unit in the middle of the night.

As a student nurse you will almost certainly enjoy good health and probably had to give some evidence of fitness before being accepted for nurse training. Part of the assessment of your health may well have entailed some check to see that your heart is in good working order. The incidence of heart disease within the United Kingdom, however, is markedly high, so it is almost certain that you have cared for someone who has a malfunctioning heart.

Bring such a person to mind and try to remember some of his problems.

CHECK ▶

Make sure you understand and investigate the following before completing the study questions in this vignette. (See key references, page 212, for guidelines. Also consult your local Health Education Department for leaflets on educating people to care for their hearts.)

1 ▶ The normal cardiac anatomy and physiology.

2 ▶ The abnormal physiology of heart function:

    (a)   Why does the left side of the heart fail?
    (b)   Why does the right side of the heart fail?

3 ▶ Factors which may cause cardiac ischaemia.

Bill Watson is 74 years old. For the past eight years he has been aware that he has a degree of heart failure caused by hypertension. At times his heart becomes very congested causing him acute discomfort. He is admitted to hospital at 3.00 a.m. in acute distress precipitated by left ventricular failure.

Before proceeding, you should ensure that you understand what this means. *It is clearly explained in Watson & Royle (1987).*

Make a list of the specific problems which you think Bill's condition may initiate.

Dyspnoea is probably Bill's main problem. He comes in not wearing his pyjama jacket because it would be too tight for him. He is clearly fighting for every breath that he takes. A second problem is orthopnoea (difficulty in breathing lying down) and for this reason Bill is sitting up in a wheelchair. Oedema is another of Bill's problems. The pulmonary oedema, which is causing his respiratory distress, will not be apparent to the eye but you may well be able to observe that Bill's ankles are swollen and that his hands are puffy.

Have you now built up a picture of what Bill looks like?

If possible, you could discuss this with your colleagues.

It may surprise you to know that William Watson, as he prefers to be called, is a High Court Judge. It is very easy to make incorrect assumptions about people when they are in distress and not wearing their normal attire.

The main aims of nursing care for this gentleman are to reduce the workload of the heart, provide a stressfully free environment, and observe the efficiency of the drug therapy being used. Nursing care plans should be devised with these objectives in mind.

Consider how you would plan care in order to meet these aims.

Mr Watson's immediate treatment will possibly be centred around drug therapy. The aims of this are to reduce stress and heart workload and if you, as a nurse, understand this, it will enable you to care more effectively for him.

To reduce stress, diamorphine will certainly be given as this relieves the dyspnoea by relieving anxiety, peripheral venous dilatation, and reducing sensitivity of the respiratory centre to the reflex stimulation from the stiff, congested lungs. Aminophylline may be given. This would be administered slowly intravenously as this lowers the venous pressure and so relieves bronchospasm. Oxygen is beneficial as congestion in Mr Watson's lungs will have caused an imbalance between ventilation and profusion. Intravenous frusemide will relieve the pulmonary, and ultimately peripheral, oedema. Digoxin may well be given intravenously also. It is also very possible that Mr Watson has been taking oral frusemide and digoxin on a daily basis at home.

In order to reduce the work-load of the heart, Mr Watson should sit upright, probably in a chair rather than in bed.

The imbalance between ventilation and perfusion may have led to his becoming very cyanosed or he may even be coughing up frothy sputum.

Reduction of stress is essential. There can be few situations more frightening than that where it is difficult to breathe. An explanation to Mr Watson of the cause of his problem and exactly what you are going to do about it will help (*see* further student activity).

Pulmonary oedema should be relieved by the diuretic therapy but peripheral oedema may prove more persistent and may well cause discomfort. Areas particularly affected are likely to be the hands and the feet, so it is advisable to ensure that Mr Watson is not wearing rings or slippers which could become increasingly tight. There may be an oedematous area at the base of the spine; ensure that Mr Watson is sitting comfortably and well supported by pillows. The scrotum can also become uncomfortably oedematous, and it may help Mr Watson to wear a scrotum support for a short period.

The problems that Mr Watson is having with breathing may well have left a dryness of the mouth so you should make sure that he can easily reach water or a mouthwash. A sputum pot should be placed within arm's length as he is coughing up a lot of sputum. It really is important to keep a clean sputum pot at hand as he may initially fill pots up very quickly.

Hopefully the diuretic effect will very soon become apparent. Mr Watson may be more comfortable sitting on a commode, and a nurse should be ready to help him to do this if he wishes. Otherwise a urinal should be within reaching distance.

In contrast, on the same night, Graham Dawson is admitted. He has just celebrated his 65th bithday and retirement from work. He suffers from acute myocardial infarction.

Before continuing, make sure that you understand exactly what these words mean. *The referenced books by Watson & Royle (1987) and Henderson (1980) will help.*

Try now to contrast the disease process in Mr Watson's heart with that which has occurred in Mr Dawson's heart.

Mr Watson has a chronic condition which 'flares up' and causes him great discomfort. Mr Dawson has had an acute, unpremeditated attack caused by a blockage of a vessel which should normally supply the heart with blood.

When the heart becomes congested, as in Mr Watson's case, it cannot pump blood adequately so that, in time, the lung also becomes congested. In Mr Dawson's situation, necrosis of the myocardium has occurred, possibly as a result of coronary artery occlusion. Myocardial infarction can precipitate left ventricular dysfunction which in the long term may lead to pulmonary congestion.

Using the references provided identify the specific problems which Mr Dawson may experience on admission.

The overriding symptom which Mr Dawson will experience will almost certainly be a crushing chest pain, which may radiate into both arms or towards the neck or lower jaw. The pain may be accompanied by nausea, vomiting, sweating, palpitations and, almost certainly, marked anxiety.

If Mr Dawson's blood pressure is very low this could be associated with low cardiac output which may well lead to cardiogenic shock. He may also have a slight pyrexia with a temperature of about 38 degrees centigrade, but it's unlikely that it will go any higher.

Treatment for Mr Watson was centred around easing his breathing. What will the main focus of treatment for Mr Dawson be?

Try to identify the main aim for yourself.

The main aim immediately will be to reduce the extreme pain which Mr Dawson is experiencing. To do this will reduce the possibility of shock occurring. Morphine sulphate may be administered. This will almost certainly be given intravenously and nursing care must be aimed at monitoring respirations as this drug can cause depression of the respiratory centre.

Oxygen will probably be administered as this, too, will help to reduce the pain which results from hypoxia and it may also help to prevent the infarction from spreading.

How will nursing care be managed to meet Mr Dawson's needs at this time?

Nursing care will be centred around resting Mr Dawson and relieving his anxiety. Both of these measures should help to reduce his pain and his breathing problem. He will probably be most comfortable sitting at an angle of about 45° in a semi-recumbent position, as this position allows for greater lung expansion.

Mr Dawson will certainly be attached to an electro-cardiogram monitor.

Do you feel anxious about caring for someone attached to a cardiac monitor? If so, think how much more anxious Mr Dawson will feel. What will you say to help him at this time?

Any of the following references may be of use to you here: Gardiner 1981, Hubner 1980 and Thompson 1986.

It should be explained to Mr Dawson and his family that the monitor is a means of getting a constant picture of the action of his heart. It is not treating him or affecting his heart in any way. To nurse a patient who is having his heart monitored effectively, you should make sure you understand what a normal ECG tracing looks like (*see* further student activity).

Mr Dawson makes a steady recovery. His chest pain lasts for two to three hours by which time the cardiac monitor is giving evidence of a heart which is in sinus rhythm. His skin, which had been moist and grey, owing to the degree of cardiac output, returns to its normal colouring. However, he does remain very tired and understandably anxious.

A gradual day-by-day programme of mobilization is implemented for him.

Mrs Dawson is extremely anxious. She is terrified about her husband coming home, she feels very uncertain about how to care for him and is worried about their future lives together. Mr Dawson's tiredness persists and he cannot concentrate for long periods of time. He seems very depressed and even tearful on occasions.

Try to design a good specific discharge plan which will help both Mr and Mrs Dawson come to terms with what has happened, and how they can plan their future lives.

References to Roper, Logan and Tierney (1985) will help here.

Drawing up such a plan may take some time, but it should be done in conjunction with the patient. In fact it should be the patient's plan.

It may be beneficial to consider the activities of daily living and formulate a plan around these. For example, when looking at mobility you could consider just exactly how far Mr Dawson should walk each day in terms of *Day 1* – walk to the bottom of the garden and back; *Day 2* – walk to the sweet shop; *Day 3* – walk up to the park.

When talking about work, rest and play, you should try to find out how Mr Dawson normally spends his leisure time and make a specific plan of care in relation to that. If he is a golf player, for instance, you could between you work out the point at which it would be sensible for him to try to play a round of golf. Of course, Mr Dawson should be made aware that if he experiences any pain, discomfort, or difficulty in breathing then he should reduce the amount that he is doing each day and contact his doctor.

Once a detailed plan has been drawn up, you should ensure that both Mr Dawson and his wife understand it by asking them to explain it fully to you. See that they have a written copy to take home with them as this will reinforce the information. It's surprising how much security a piece of paper can give.

It would be beneficial for you to elaborate on this care plan. *A most useful reference here is Elwes & Simnett (1985).*

SUMMARY AND FURTHER STUDY

We have considered the needs of two men, each of whom has a malfunctioning heart but whose needs are somewhat different. In the case of each it is essential that he should feel confident enough to carry on a full, normal, life-style. Careful planning for discharge home will help these two men to achieve this aim.

1 Both Mr Dawson and Mr Watson are fairly obese. How, as the health educator, would you explain to them the need to lose weight in order to reduce the blood pressure?

2 Having done this, how would you impress upon them the need to monitor cholesterol intake, and reduce, if not cut out, cigarette smoking?

3 Draw the PQRST segment of a normal electro-cardiogram. Indicate what is happening to the heart at each stage on the diagram.

REFERENCES TO VIGNETTE 21

KEY REFERENCES

Henderson, I. 1980. *Heart Attacks Understood*. Macmillan, London.

Holmes, H. E. 1983. A question of sport. (Does exercise reduce heart disease?) *Nursing Times Mirror*, 25 February, pp.19–20.

Llunt, D. 1985. Cardiac failure. *Nursing Mirror*, 22 May, pp.41–2.

McCulloch, J. 1985. *Focus on Coronary Care*. Heinemann, London. Nursing Mirror. 1983. Too young to die (A description of a heart attack by a 29-year-old nurse). *Nursing Mirror*, 156(22), 21 June, pp.46–7.

Watson, J. E. and Royle, R. J. 1987. *Watson's Medical-Surgical Nursing and Related Physiology*. 3rd edition. Baillière Tindall, London.

ADDITIONAL REFERENCES

Elwes, L. and Simnett, J. 1985. *Promoting Health. A Practical Guide to Health Education*. John Wiley & Sons, London.

Gardiner, J. 1981. *The ECG. What Does It Mean?* Stanley Thornes, London.

Hubner, P. 1980. *Nurses' Guide to Cardiac Monitoring*. Baillière Tindall, London.

Thompson, D. 1986. Patients' views on cardiac monitoring. *Nursing Times & Mirror*, 82, pp.54–5.

Roper, N., Logan, W. W. and Tierney, A. J. 1985. *The Elements of Nursing*, 2nd edition. Churchill Livingstone, Edinburgh.

ROSE WILKINS

Rose is dying in hospital.

Helping a person achieve a peaceful death is a worthwhile aim of nursing care, and encountered often in the daily practice of nurses. It is especially challenging because care and concern is also directed towards the dying person's friends and relatives.

Bring to mind the dying people you have nursed.

What did you learn during these experiences?

What do you consider to be the most important goals of care for these patients?

CHECK ▶   Make sure you understand and investigate the following before completing the study questions in the vignette (see key references, page 216, for helpful literature):

1 ▶   The principles of the nursing and medical care of a person with pneumonia.

2 ▶   The principles of nursing the dying and promoting their comfort and dignity.

Rose Wilkins is 86 years old. She lives in a warden-controlled residential housing complex, in a one-bedroomed flat. Mrs Wilkins was a milliner and a housewife in her working life. Up until recently she was a willing baby sitter and baked marvellous cakes for all sorts of occasions for her large and loving family.

Two years age she fell and fractured her neck of femur; she recovered some of her mobility but began to lose confidence in herself and her capabilities. Recently Mrs Wilkins developed a chest infection and eventually felt unable to get up one morning. The warden called in her GP and Mrs Wilkins' eldest daughter, May. Mrs Wilkins had pneumonia and according to the doctor needed to be treated with antibiotics, oxygen therapy, physiotherapy and nursing.

May wanted her mother to have the best treatment possible and did not feel that she could really care for her as well as hospital personnel could, and yet she felt unsure as to what would be best.

Mrs Wilkins herself was feverish and kept asking where Alf was – Alfred Wilkins, her husband, had died ten years previously, and this rather unnerved May.

The doctor explained to Mrs Wilkins that she was going to be taken to hospital so that she could have a rest and get better. She was dozing off to sleep and did not seem to mind. May packed a small suitcase of items for use in hospital and accompanied her mother in the ambulance when it arrived later in the morning.

As soon as she arrived on a medical ward Mrs Wilkins had an intravenous infusion started and her first dose of a broad spectrum antibiotic was given intravenously. She was prescribed oxygen therapy by means of a mask which delivered 60 per cent concentration to correct her hypoxia, and intravenous fluids to correct her dehydration.

Given the information so far, write a care plan outlining the way in which Mrs Wilkins will be nursed for the next 24 hours.

Write down the specific criteria you would use to decide whether the care given had been effective.

Mrs Wilkins is a well-loved grandmother and great-grandmother. Her granddaughter Jean, May's daughter, a trained nurse, asks that evening to be allowed, with her mother, to help care for Mrs Wilkins.

How can Jean and her mother be supported in their desire to help nurse Mrs Wilkins?

What benefits can you envisage will develop as a result of enabling Mrs Wilkins' relatives to assist with her nursing care?

Two days later Mrs Wilkins remains confused. She had pulled out her intravenous cannula twice and would not accept wearing an oxygen mask. She remained slightly pyrexial and breathless. The ward sister and the nurses caring for Mrs Wilkins arranged a meeting with May and Jean to discuss her care. Together they talked about what sort of person Mrs Wilkins was and one particular dimension, her spiritual nature, came to the forefront of the discussion. It seemed quite possible that Mrs Wilkins would not recover from the pneumonia and since she seemed so distressed it was felt that this could be an important area of care to focus on. The ward sister asked Reverend Sheila Goode, the hospital chaplain, to see Mrs Wilkins and her family.

This dimension of patient care may be one where you are uncertain about your role. Resources you can consult include McGilloway and Myco 1985, Neuberger 1987 and Sampson 1982.

Other dimensions of care were discussed, and May and Jean, together with the ward staff, felt that Mrs Wilkins' care, given that she was dying, should be directed towards ensuring her comfort. Although May had felt some misgivings about her mother going into hospital initially, she did not feel that there would be any great benefit for herself or her mother in transferring her home. The staff assured May and Jean that their involvement in Mrs Wilkins' care was welcome. At the meeting the ward staff also discussed whether Mrs Wilkins should be moved from the ten-bedded ward into a single room.

For a study on whether people want to die at home, and the role of the family in their care see Woodhall 1986.

What factors would you take into account in reaching a decision about this matter?

Mrs Wilkins' needs for care were reassessed at this point.

What readjustments would you make to Mrs Wilkins' care plan, taking into account the present situation?

During the next few days Mrs Wilkins slept for short periods during the day and night. However, when she was awake she became distressed, agitated and breathless. She was not calm enough to be able to drink and eat. She was prescribed sub-cutaneous injections of diamorphine to relieve this distress and breathlessness.

During a coffee break in the hospital canteen, two student nurses are discussing Mrs Wilkins' care. Imagine you are the senior of the two. The other nurse, a first ward nurse, tells you that she does not agree with what is 'going on' with Mrs Wilkins and will not act as a witness to the administration of the diamorphine as she feels it is unethical. 'They are just killing her off.'

Think through how you could help her to explore the morality of giving opiate drugs in this sort of situation.

By the end of the week Mrs Wilkins was sleeping for most of the time. Her breathing was rapid and shallow but she was quite calm and not distressed. Her breathing was noisy and worried Jean and May, and so hyoscine was added to the diamorphine injections which minimized the respiratory secretions and made her breathing less noisy.

Refocus your attention on May and Jean. One or other of them is always present during the day and late into the evening.

How can they be cared for by the ward team at this point?

Mrs Wilkins is repositioned every two hours and her mouth is cleaned and moistened. She has a urinary catheter to prevent the discomfort of being incontinent. When she is repositioned, and at other times if she is awake, she is helped to sip some lemon barley water or some apple juice, which are her favourite soft drinks. She has not received any significant nourishment for almost a week although she is still receiving fluids by means of an intravenous infusion which does not disturb her, and which May and Jean have asked to be continued. Her spiritual care is continued and the Rector of her local church visits and prays with her and for her.

Mrs Wilkins has lived in a way which reflects her Christian beliefs and she has been an active church member throughout her life. Her relatives and the nurses caring for her are enabling her to maintain these religious practices which seem to comfort her. Nursing research is increasingly focusing on this area of patient care (see Simsen 1986).

DISCUSSION AND FURTHER STUDY

1 Rose Wilkins is dying peacefully in a general medical ward where nurses, together with her relatives, are achieving care which promotes her comfort and maintains her dignity. To help a person die peacefully in hospital wards can be difficult, and you may be familiar with these difficulties. An investigation of this issue can be found in Hockley (1983).

2 The experiences of people who are dying has been explored in Kubler-Ross 1969 and Glaser and Strauss 1965.

REFERENCES TO VIGNETTE 22

KEY REFERENCES

Hector, W. and Whitfield, S. 1982. *Nursing Care for the Dying Patient and the Family*. William Heinemann, London.

Redfern, S. J. (ed.) 1986. *Nursing Elderly People*. Churchill Livingstone, Edinburgh.

Roper, N., Logan, W. L. and Tierney, A. J. 1985. *The Elements of Nursing*, 2nd edition, chs.9, 18. Churchill Livingstone, Edinburgh.

Saunders, C. M. 1978. *The Management of Terminal Diseases*. Edward Arnold, London.

ADDITIONAL REFERENCES

Glaser, B. G. and Strauss, A. 1965. *Awareness of Dying*. Aldine Publishing Co., New York.

Hockley, J. 1983. An Investigation to Identify Symptoms of Distress in the Terminally Ill Patient and Family in the General Medical Ward.

Unpublished report. St Bartholomew's Hospital. Hockley's investigations are also reported in Sadler, C. 1984. Clinical review. *Nursing Mirror*, 21 March, p.12.

Kubler-Ross, E. 1969. *On Death and Dying*. Macmillan, New York.

McGilloway, O. and Myco, F. (eds) 1985. *Nursing and Spiritual Care*. Lippincott Nursing series. Harper & Row, London.

Neuberger, J. 1987. *Caring for Dying People of Different Faiths*. Austen Cornish , London.

Sampson, C. 1982. *The Neglected Ethic: Religious and Cultural Factors in the Care of Patients*. McGraw-Hill (U.K.) Ltd, Maidenhead.

Simsen, B. 1986. The spiritual dimension. *Nursing Times*, 26 November, pp.41–2.

Woodhall, C. 1986. A family concern. *Nursing Times*, 22 October, pp.31–3.

DEREK WILLIAMS

Derek has diabetes mellitus and is too busy to look after his health.

Taking on the role of health educator with patients is not just a matter of nurses teaching patients how to be more healthy, or how to care for themselves when they have a health problem. It also encompasses a counselling and listening role, by which means nurses can try to help patients to deal with the reasons why, in certain circumstances, they choose not to care for themselves, even though as health professionals we might have expected them to.

Bring to mind the patients you have nursed who have diabetes mellitus.

What health education did each require, and who supplied it?

CHECK ▶ Make sure you understand and investigate the following before completing the study questions in this vignette (see key references, page 221):

1 ▶   The possible causes of the two main types of diabetes mellitus.

2 ▶   The physiological effects of uncontrolled diabetes mellitus.

3 ▶   The principal ways in which diabetes mellitus can be controlled.

Derek Williams is a sales manager for a large retailing organization which has stores in every high street throughout the country. He is responsible for the North West of England. At present he lives in a small company flat in London. He and his wife, Natalie, are separated and awaiting finalization of their divorce. She lives in the family home in the suburbs of Birmingham with their two children, Amy and Jeffrey. Over the past year Derek has immersed himself totally in his work, with rising sales figures and a substantial rise in salary to recompense him.

Last Tuesday he was found slumped over his desk by his secretary Joyce. She knew he was a diabetic and she tried to rouse him to get him to drink some sweetened fruit juice, but she did not succeed. Joyce called in the occupational health nurse who took a finger prick blood glucose test which showed that the level of Derek's blood glucose was abnormally high. Subsequently Derek was taken to hospital by ambulance in a hyperglycaemic (ketoacidotic) coma.

Outline for yourself the medical strategy for dealing with a hyperglycaemic coma.

Taking into account the medical treatment, outline the key points of the nursing assessment to be made on admission, and the immediate nursing activities which will be planned to meet Derek's needs as an unconscious patient in a hyperglycaemic coma.

An initial nursing assessment will have taken into account Derek's physiological needs. Once he becomes conscious his psycho-social and spiritual needs can be assessed and planned for.

Derek regains consciousness during the evening in response to treatment with intravenous fluids and insulin. The nurse caring for him explains what has happened to him, where he is, and what is being done to correct his condition. In response to her explanation he says, 'Mmm, I'm afraid this is all my own fault. I'm sorry.'

Write down what you think would be the 'right' response for a nurse to make to Derek's statement. Try to give specific reasons for the response you choose. (See French, 1983. The section on 'active listening' skills will be helpful.)

Derek has an ulcer on the inner aspect of his left foot just below the ankle. This is thought to have resulted from his diabetic condition.

Can you explain why Derek's ulcer is linked to his diabetes mellitus?

What other physiological changes take place over time in a person with diabetes mellitus, and what symptoms may the patient experience as a result? (See Thurston and Beattie 1984 a, b.)

Derek explains that the ulcer on his foot has been there for about four weeks. He realized it was connected to his diabetes, but felt at the time just too busy to do anything about it. Derek did not attend his last hospital outpatient appointment. At these consultations the diabetic person's health is checked and their personal recordings of the results of the blood or urine tests they perform at home, and the doses of insulin they have administered, are discussed. He was sent a letter asking him to telephone and make another appointment, but he felt too busy and too preoccupied with his work and his impending divorce to do this, and he put his own care of his health into the background.

It may seem completely reasonable to us to expect patients to accept and take action about the advice and teaching they have been given about their health, particularly if they have a health problem such as diabetes. However, it may be the case that our advice is very difficult at times to incorporate into the life-styles of many of our patients. An interesting account of the everyday reality of living with diabetes is given in Drummond 1985.

The clinical nurse specialist in diabetic care visits Derek and assesses his current needs for health teaching and counselling. She considers that he is, at this point, highly motivated to reassess his health and its value to him. (Strategies in teaching people with diabetes are discussed in Marks 1983 and Batehup 1986.)

Derek expresses interest in using a blood glucose meter, rather than in testing his urine, as he has done in the past.

For background information on this equipment and its impact on the health education of people with diabetes see Newton 1987, Hilton 1986 and Reading 1986.

What is your opinion about the patient hand-out that is outlined in the last article?

One particular aspect of Derek's working life that is presenting difficulties for him is his need, since his recent promotion, to entertain clients two or three times a week. This involves eating out and drinking alcohol. In order to accommodate to this change in his life-style Derek is going to need information, and he will need the assistance of the dietician, the doctor and the clinical nurse specialist.

Investigate for yourself the principles that underlie the nutrition of a person with diabetes. (See patient education materials used in your hospital, and Faulkner 1985.)

DISCUSSION AND FURTHER STUDY

Derek Williams has undergone a health crisis which has been resolved. It has provided him with an opportunity to reassess the importance or otherwise he has attached to caring for his health. In his situation, the nurse's role as a health educator has been predominantly one of listening to him and allowing him to make his own health choices. The circumstances of his personal and professional life mean that he needs to think through how he can further adjust to having diabetes and to the limits it places on his life-style.

1 Derek Williams is almost at the peak of his career. His success has had repercussions on his personal relationships. He is reassessing his life at this point, early middle age. For a discussion of the developmental needs of people at this time see Sheehy 1977.

2 For a discussion of the developments in the medical care of people with diabetes see Dinsdale and Cochrane 1986 and Medows 1984.

3 People with diabetes can gain practical help and support by being put in touch with a self-help organization such as the British Diabetic Association. A brief description of its work is given in Noakes 1984.

4 This vignette has highlighted the role of nurses in the care of people with diabetes. Two nurses have important roles alongside Derek Williams; the occupational health nurse in his place of work, and the clinical nurse specialist for diabetic care, based at his local hospital. Both may be involved with his care by counselling and supporting him, and by helping him monitor his diabetes.

A leading article in the *Lancet* (1982) discusses the role of nurses in this field. What is your opinion about this article?

REFERENCES TO VIGNETTE 23

KEY REFERENCES

Faulkner, A. 1985. *Nursing. A Creative Approach*. Baillière Tindall, London.

Gill, G. V. and Alberti, K. G. 1985. Management of diabetic ketoacidosis. *Practical Diabetes*, 2(2), March/April, pp.12–16.

Reading, S. 1986. What is diabetes? *Professional Nurse*, 1(12), September, pp.333–4.

ADDITIONAL REFERENCES

Batehup, L. 1986. Helping a patient understand diabetes. *Nursing Times*, 19 March, pp.46–9.

Dinsdale, C. and Cochrane, W. 1986. The changing face for treatment of diabetes. *Nursing Times*, 12 February, pp.36–7.

Drummond, N. 1985. Against doctor's orders. *New Society*, 4 October, pp.11–12.

French, P. 1983. *Social Skills for Nursing Practice*. Croom Helm, London.

Hilton, A. 1986. Nursing practice. Monitoring blood glucose levels. *Nursing Times*, 30 April, pp.55–6.

Lancet. 1982. The place of nurses in management of diabetes. *Lancet*, 16 January, pp.145–6.

Marks, C. 1983. Teaching the diabetic patient. In Wilson-Barnett, J. (ed.) *Patient Teaching*. Churchill Livingstone, Edinburgh.

Medows, S. 1984. Insulin without tears. *Nursing Times*, 22 August, pp.40–2.

Newton, R. 1987. Testing, testing . . . *Nursing Times*, Community Outlook Supplement, 14 January, pp.16–18.

Noakes, B. 1984. Helping diabetics help themselves. *Nursing Times*, 22 August, pp.46–8.

Reading, S. 1986. Blood glucose monitoring: teaching effective techniques. *Professional Nurse*, 2(2), November, pp.55–7.

Sheehy, G. 1977. *Passages: Predictable Crises of Adult Life*. Bantam Books, New York.

Thurston, R. and Beattie, C. 1984a. Foot lesions in diabetes. Predisposing factors. *Nursing Times*, 22 August, pp.44–6.

Thurston, R. and Beattie, C. 1984b. Foot lesions in diabetes: care of a patient. *Nursing Times*, 29 August, pp.48–50.

INDEX

abortions 202–06
accident victims, nursing 143–4
accidents, liability for 92–3
action research 68
Action for Research into Multiple Sclerosis 131
activities of living 28–9
acute lymphoblastic leukemia 182
Addison's disease 195
adolescence, psychology 152
adrenal glands 192, 193, 195
adrenalectomy 195
adulthood 162
affective components, ethics 84
Afro-Caribbeans, sickle cell trait 189
ageing 116
agency nurses 140
aggression, patients confined to bed 165
Aid for Down's Babies 106
aides 36
AIDS 137–140, 195
AIDS-related complex 137
alcohol, legal limit in bloodstream 147
Alcohol Studies Centre 147, 150
allergic reactions, cystitis 172, 173
Alzheimer's disease 99–102
aminophylline 208
amputation, lower limbs 142–6
anaemia 187, 190
analysis, experimental data 69–73
anger, bereavement 148
anti-inflammatory drugs 124
antibiotics 134, 139, 188
antibody formation 137
anxiety, cancer patients 111
aplastic anaemia 190
appendicectomy, emergency 134
appendix, ruptured 133–5
arterial circulation 142
aspirin 124
assessment, nursing process 26–7, 30, 31, 100
at risk register 157, 159–60
audit, nursing records 35
awareness, lack of, stroke patients 118

babies
  physical activities 157–8
  sickle cell trait 189
bacteria, cystitis 172, 173
Bangladeshis 205
bar charts, data presentation 72–3
bed confinement, lengthy 162–6
behaviour, Alzheimer's disease 99–100
behavioural components, ethics 84
bereavement 147

Bergman's ethical decision-making model 91–2, 204
Block Report 44
bladder infection 170, 172
blood glucose levels 219
blood glucose meters 220
blood tests 183
blood transfusion 188
body image 192–5
bone marrow 182
bone marrow aspirations 183
bone marrow transplants 185
books 20–1
  use of 19–20
bowel preparation, pre-operative 198
breast cancer 177–80, 195
breast self-examination 178
breast surgery 177, 178, 179
British Diabetic Association 220
British Rheumatism and Arthritis Association 126
broken bones, healing 162
bronchoscopy 110, 111
bronchus, squamous cell carcinoma 111

cancer, breast 177–80, 195
cancer, lung 110–14
cancer patients, nursing 114
carcinogenesis 110
cardiac ischaemia 207
cardiac units 207–12
care
  post-operative 144–5
  terminally ill 113–14
care plans 32
  dying patients 215–16
  pneumonia 214
  pre-operative 198
  stroke patients 117
  writing 36
care of property, disclaiming of responsibility 93
carers
  dependent relatives 101
  spouses 125–6
causes, lung cancer 110
central nervous system 128–9
cerebrovascular accidents 116, 117
chaplains 214
chemotherapy 180
chest infection 213
chest pain 210
child abuse 157–60
child abuse register 159
child development 104, 107, 157, 183
childhood 162
children
  Down's syndrome 104–8

in hospital 183
leukemia 182–5
cholesterol intake, monitoring 212
chromosomes, Down's syndrome 105
chronic leukemia 185
cigarette smoking 110, 143, 212
class, health inequality and 44–5
clinical nurse specialists 179, 221
co-trimoxazole 139
code of conduct, UKCC 92
cognitive components, ethics 84
communication
  with non-English speakers 134, 135
  nurse-patient 200
communication skills, nurses 51–2, 62
community nurses 113, 120
competencies, registered nurses 17–18, 25
concurrent audit, nursing records 35
consent, medical treatment 93–4
constipation 164
control groups, experiments 65, 68
counselling
  after pregnancy termination 205
  mastectomy patients 179
critical questions, research reports 75–8
cross-infection 139, 200
Cruse 149
crutches 145
curriculum, nursing 17–18
Curtin's ethical decision-making model 89–91, 204
custodialism, nursing ideology 30
cystitis 169–75
cytotoxic drugs 178, 180, 183, 184

daily living, activities of 28–9, 131
data
  analysis and evaluation 69–73
  collection, research 65–9
death 147–50
decision-making
  ethical dilemmas 89–92
  ethics 86–7, 94–5, 165
  nursing process 26–7
dehydration 137
dementia, elderly 99–102
denial, bereavement 148
dental hygiene 48
dependence, drugs 152
dependent relatives, carers 101
depression 193
descriptive research 68
design, research 65–9
diabetes mellitus 195, 218–21

diagnosis 47
  cancer 111
  Down's syndrome 104
diamorphine 215
diet
  elderly people 119
  Hindus 135
digoxin 208
diomorphine 208
disabled children, education services 106
Disabled Living Foundation 125, 130, 131
discharge plans, heart patients 210, 212
diuretic therapy 209
doctor-induced disease 46
doctors
  consulting 45
  cystitis treatment 174–5
Down's Children's Association 106
Down's syndrome 104–8
drinking and driving 147, 150
drug abuse 156
drug addiction 152
drug therapy, rheumatoid arthritis 124
drugs, misuse 152
duties 86
duty-based theories, ethics 86, 87
dying 213–16
  at home 215
dysarthia 118
dysponoea 208

eating, healthy 50, 51
eating habits, elderly people 119
economic constraints, long-term illness 130
economic factors, affecting health 44–5
education, handicapped children 108
education services, disabled children 106
elderly people
  dementia 99–102
  falls 100
  stroke 116–20
electro-cardiogram monitors 210–11
emdocrine disorders 195
emotional health 42, 43
emotions, parents with handicapped children 105
empirical research 67–8
endocrine disorder 192–5
environment, health and 43
ethical dilemmas 87–9, 108, 123
  strategies for resolving 89–92
ethics

in nursing practice 83–92, 190, 204, 215
research projects 75
ethnic minority groups
health needs 190
nursing 133–5
sickle cell trait 189
euthanasia 114
evaluation
experimental data 69–73
nursing process 26–7, 30, 33
research 79
exercise, fractured femur 165
experimental groups 65, 68
experimental research 68
eye care, rheumatoid arthritis 124–5

facts, collecting, in research 63
falls, elderly people 100
families
AIDS patients 139–40
dying patients 215
effects of Down's Syndrome 107–8
family planning, advice 205
fasting, pre-operative 198
female urinary tract 169
femur, fracture 99, 162–6
financial help, multiple sclerosis 130
first aid, cystitis 170–1
fluoridation, water supply 48
foetal development 202, 203
folic acid 124
foot lesions, diabetes 219
Forest Report 180
fracture, femur 99, 162–6
friction, cystitis 172, 173
frusemide 208
funding, research 74–5

general practitioners 113, 203
germs, cystitis 172, 173
glue sniffing 152–6
goals 86
government agencies, support for Down's syndrome parents 105–7
graphs, data presentation 71–2
grief 105, 147, 148, 150, 205
guilt, pregnancy termination 204
haemoglobin 187
haemolytic anaemia 190
haemorrhage, post-operative 204
handicapped children, education 108
healing
broken bones 162
post-operative 199
health
detrimental situations 41
economic and social factors 44–5
meaning of 41–3
promotion 41
responsibility for 43
health advice, nurses 169

health authorities, quality assurance programmes 35
health education 48, 195, 212
diabetes mellitus 218, 220
health educators, nurses as 49–51, 175
health services, use of 46
health visitors 106–7, 108, 120
healthy living, nurses as role models for 51–2
heart, anatomy and physiology 207
heart disease 207–12
helping relationship, nurse-patient 29–30
hemiplegia, left-sided 117, 118
heritability, sickle cell disease 189
hernia 197
herpes 173
Hickman catheters 183
Hindus 134, 135
hip replacement 124
historical research 68
HIV 137
hormone balance, alteration 178
hospices 113, 114
hospital chaplains 214
Human Immunodeficiency Virus 137, 139
hygiene
AIDS 139
patients confined to bed 165
hyperglycaemic comas 219
hypertension 207
hypothermia 117
hypotheses, in research 63–5
hypothyroidism 189
hypoxia 187

iatrogenesis 46
Ibuprofen 124
idealogies, nursing 30
ill health
developing 45–6
prevention 47–9
illness
established, minimizing effects 48
prevention 41
immunity 137
immunization 48
immuno-suppressant drugs 124
implementation, nursing process 26–7, 30, 32
incidence, lung cancer 110
incontinence 118, 129
individualized care 30
infections
leukemia patients 184
non-bacterial 173
information, gathering 61–2
inguinal hernia 197–200
initial planning options 32
injuries, accidents 143–4
intellectual skills, children 183
interviews, research 67
intravenous fluids 134, 188
intuitionalism 86, 87

inverse care law 46
iron deficiency anaemia 190
ischaemia 142, 143

journals, use of 19–20

labelling, health problems 47
language remediation programmes 107
learning difficulties, severe 107
left ventricular dysfunction 209
left ventricular failure 207–9
legal issues, nursing 92–5, 204
legs, amputation 142–6
leukemia, children 182–5
liability, for accidents 92–3
libraries, use of 19–20
life-style, diabetes and 220
liquids, in cystitis 171, 173
living, activities of 28–9
lower limbs, amputation 142–6
lung cancer 110–14

macrocytic anaemia 124
mammography 178
mastectomy 177
Mastectomy Association 179
meals-on-wheel's service 120
media, reports of child abuse 157
medical diagnosis 47
medical treatment, consent 93–4
mental health 42, 43
metastases 110, 112
breast cancer 180
micturition, control 118
middle age 220
miscarriage 203
models, nursing 25, 26–7
moral philosophy 83–7
mouth care, rheumatoid arthritis 124–5
movement, fractured femur 165
mutliple sclerosis 128–31
Multiple Sclerosis Society of Great Britain and Northern Ireland 131
muscle, necrosis 143
Muslims 205
myocardial infarction 209–11

necrosis, muscle 143
neutropaenic patients 184
Norton Score 60
notes 21
NSPCC 159–160
null hypothesis 64–5, 65
nurse-patient relationship 29–30
nurses
competencies 17–18, 25
as health educators 49–51, 175
as role models for healthy living 51–2
nursing
cancer patients 114
concept of 27–9
ethical issues 83–92, 190, 204
history of research in 59–60
ideologies 30

legal issues 92–5, 204
models 25, 26–7
politics of 36
post-operative 195
primary 33–4
relevance of research 60–1
research 57–9, 61–72
studying 19–21
team 33
nursing assessment 26–7, 30, 31, 100
AIDS 138
diabetes mellitus 219
endocrine disorder 193–4
lung cancer 112–13
multiple sclerosis 131
stroke patients 117–18
nursing care
delivering 33–4
fractured femur 99
left ventricular failure 208
management 25–36
measuring quality 34–6
myocardial infarction 210
nursing education 17–18
nursing history, rheumatoid arthritis 122
nursing intervention, patients confined to bed 164–5
nursing process 25, 30–3
decision-making 26–7
nutrition 50–51
diabetes 220
elderly people 119, 120

obesity, heart patients 212
obligations, patients 47
observational learning 51
occupational health nurses 221
occupational therapists 166
operations, patients reactions to 143
oral hygiene, AIDS 139
orthopaedic wards 166
orthopnoea 208
osteo-arthrosis 122, 123
outcome, nursing care 35
oxygen therapy 139, 188, 214

paediatric wards 182
PAIN 159
pain 163
after myocardial infarction 210
assessment and relief 188
cystitis 171
post-operative 199
parents 165
children with leukemia 183, 185
solvent abuse and 153–4
patient allocation 33
patients
consent to medical treatment 93–4
demanding 125
dying 213–16
expectations of 47
needs 25
nursing assessment 31

self-caring 28
people, consulting 19
peripheral oedema 209
peripheral vascular disease 142,
 143
pernicious anaemia 190
personal ethic 85
personal experience, reflection
 on 20
personal responsibility, for health
 43
personality, Alzheimer's disease
 99–100
persons, respect for 52
phenylketonuria 189
philosophical research 68–9
physical activities, babies and
 toddlers 157–8
physical problems, prolonged bed
 confinement 163–4
physical skills, children 183
physiological aspects, ageing 116
physiotherapists 166
pilot studies, research 67
pins and needles, multiple
 sclerosis 129
planning, nursing process 26–7,
 30, 32
platelets 182, 183, 184
playgroups 107
pleural effusion 112, 113
pneumonia 137, 139, 213
politics of nursing 36
post-operative care 101
 termination of pregnancy 204–5
pre-operative care 134
pre-operative preparation,
 mastectomy 179
pregnancy, termination 202–5
premedication 199
prevention
 cystitis 173–4
 lung cancer 110
 solvent abuse 155
primary health care teams 113
primary nursing 33–4
 children's wards 184
primary prevention, ill health 48
privacy, lack of 163
privileges, patients 47
probability 73
problem, identification, in
 research 63
process, nursing care 35
profession, nursing ideology 30
professional ethic 85–6
profusion 208, 209
property, care of 93
prostheses, lower limb 144, 145
psychology

adolescence 152
ageing 116
pulmonary oedema 208

quality assurance programmes 35
questionnaires, research 67

radiation treatment, breast cancer
 180
radiographers 166
radiotherapy 111, 177, 178, 179,
 180, 184
random sampling 66
Rastafarians 205
red blood cells 182, 187
reflection, on personal
 experience 20
registered nurses, competencies
 17–18
rehabilitation, post-operative
 144–5
religion
 dying patients 215
 ethics and 84–5
renal system 172
reporting, research 73–5
research 57–9
 funding 74–5
 history of 59–60
 relevance 60–1
 stages 61–72
research design, critical
 questions 77
research problems, critical
 questions 76–7
research projects, ethics 75
research reports, reading 75–8
resentment, bereavement 148
resources, Down's syndrome
 patients 107
respite care 122–6
rest, cystitis 171–2
results, research 77–8
retrospective audit, nursing
 records 35
reverse barrier nursing 184
rheumatism 123
rheumatoid arthritis 122–6
rights 86
rights-based theories, ethics 86,
 87
road traffic accidents, death
 147–50
role models, nurses as 51–2

Salazopyrin 124
scatter diagrams, data
 presentation 70–1
scientific research 60
screening

breast cancer 180
 secondary prevention 48
 sickle cell trait 189
secondary prevention, ill health
 48
self-assessment, cancer patients
 114
self-caring, patients 28
self-image, developing 163
settling down, arthritic patients
 123–4
severe learning difficulties 107
sexual abuse, children 160
sexual intercourse, cystitis 173
sexual morality 205
Sexual Problems of the Disabled
 131
sexuality 192, 195
sexually transmitted diseases
 173, 174–5
sickle cell crisis 187–90
sickle cell disease 187, 189
Sickle Cell Society 189
sickle cell trait 187, 189, 190
signs, child abuse 158
Sikhs 205
skeleton traction 162, 166–7
skin preparation, pre-operative
 198
smoking 50, 51, 110, 143, 212
social aspects, ageing 116
social factors, affecting health
 44–5
social health 42–43
Social Services Departments 106
social skills, children 183
social triggers, visiting surgery 45
social workers 101, 166
society, health and 43
sodium bicarbonate, cystitis 171
solvent abuse 152–6
solvents, methods of inhalation
 154
speech, stroke patients 117
spinal cord, structure 128
spiritual health 42, 43
splints, rheumatoid arthritis 123,
 124
spontaneous abortion 203
spouses
 bereavement 148–9
 carers 125–6
 multiple sclerosis patients 129,
 130
squamous cell carcinoma 111
statistics 69, 73
steroid drugs 195
 side-effects 192
strategic nursing care, AIDS 138
stroke, elderly people 116–20

structure, nursing card 34
study resources, personal 20–1
studying, nursing 19–21
support workers 36
surgery
 consent to 134
 fractured femur 99
 inguinal hernia 197
 routine 197–200
synovial joints 122

tables, data presentation 69–70
task allocation 33
teaching, patients 49–51
teaching plans, for sickle cell
 disease 189
team nursing 33
Terence Higgins Trust 140
terminally ill, care of 113–14
tertiary prevention, ill health 48
Therapeutic Abortion Act 1967
 202, 203, 204
thrush 173
thyroid glands 195
toddlers, physical activities 157–8
tolerance, drug misuse 152
total patient care 33
toxaemia 143
trauma, amputation and 143
treatment
 leukemia 185
 lung cancer 110, 112
trichomonas 173

UKCC Code of Conduct 92
ulcers, diabetes mellitus 219
urethritis 170
urinary retention 164
urinary tract, female 169
urine, constitution 169
utilitarianism 86, 87

vaginal infections 173
variables, in experiments 65–6
ventilation 208, 209
vignettes 21–2, Part 2
vision, blurred, multiple sclerosis
 129
vocation, nursing ideology 30

washing, patients confined to bed
 165
well-being, detrimental situations
 41
white blood cells 182, 183
wills, witnessing 93
withdrawal effects, drugs 152
written consent, to medical
 treatment 94
written material, consulting 19–20